Trends in Wound Care

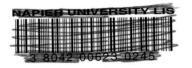

Also available from Quay Books, MA Healthcare Limited

Trends in Wound Care, volume I edited by Richard White

Trends in Wound Care
volume II

edited by
Richard J White

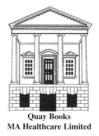

Quay Books
MA Healthcare Limited

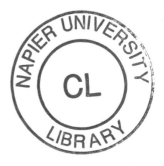

Quay Books Division, MA Healthcare Limited, Jesses Farm, Snow Hill, Dinton, Salisbury, Wiltshire, SP3 5HN

British Library Cataloguing-in-Publication Data
A catalogue record is available for this book

© MA Healthcare Limited 2003
ISBN 1 85642 246 1

Printed in Singapore by Imago

Contents

List of contributors

Jane Board is Lymphoedema Nurse Specialist, The South Bucks Day Hospice, High Wycombe, Buckinghamshire.

Pam Cooper is Clinical Nurse Specialist — Tissue Viability, Department of Tissue Viability, Aberdeen Royal Infirmary.

Tony Fowler is Customer Services Manager, Biosurgical Research Unit, Surgical Materials Testing Laboratory, Princess of Wales Hospital, Bridgend.

David Gray is Clinical Nurse Specialist — Tissue Viability, Department of Tissue Viability, Aberdeen Royal Infirmary.

Wendy Harlow is Clinical Effectiveness Facilitator, Worthing and Southlands NHS Trust, Worthing Hospital, Worthing, West Sussex.

Mary Jones is Senior Research Nurse, Biosurgical Research Unit, Surgical Materials Testing Laboratory, Princess of Wales Hospital, Bridgend.

Mark O'Brien is Clinical Nurse Specialist — Tissue Viability, Great Ormond Street Hospital, London.

Jacqueline Reilly is National Healthcare Associated Infection Surveillance Nurse Coordinator, Scottish Centre for Infection and Environmental Health, Glasgow.

Linda Russell is Tissue Viability Nurse Specialist, Queen's Hospital NHS Trust, Burton upon Trent, Staffordshire.

Elizabeth Scanlon is Nurse Consultant — Tissue Viability, Leeds North West Primary Care Trust, Leeds.

Kate Springett is Senior Lecturer in Podiatry, School of Health Professions, University of Brighton.

Nikki Stubbs is Tissue Viability Nurse Specialist, Leeds North West Primary Care Trust, St Mary's House, Leeds.

Stephen Thomas is Director, Biosurgical Research Unit, Surgical Materials Testing Laboratory, Princess of Wales Hospital, Bridgend.

Rachael Walsh is District Nurse on sabbatical from Central Manchester Primary Care Trust.

Richard J White is a Clinical Research Consultant and Medical Writer, Cornwall.

Karen Wynn is Production Manager, Biosurgical Research Unit, Surgical Materials Testing Laboratory, Princess of Wales Hospital, Bridgend.

Foreword

Dr Richard White and colleagues have built on the successful tradition in volume one of this series to bring current issues of wound care to the dedicated wound care professional. This issue interprets several current issues in wound care to help you integrate the new evidence base into everyday patient care and to make a significant difference in the lives of our patients.

Wounds are an international issue and as caregivers we face similar challenges across the globe. Under the expert editorship of Dr Richard White, a team of experts will both challenge our current knowledge base and expand the comprehension and application of new concepts to advanced wound caring.

We are all faced with the difficult task of assessing and classifying wounds. Gray, White and Cooper reassess colour differentiation as a clinical decision-making method of assisting non-specialized nurses and other healthcare professionals. The spectrum presented from black to pink is not oversimplified but can be used in conjunction with the wound infection continuum to classify and effectively manage wounds. Infection is usually diagnosed clinically, based on signs and symptoms. Bacterial swabs can be used to identify pathogens and antimicrobial sensitivity but this diagnostic test only interprets and does not diagnose infection. In this chapter, Richard White clarifies the concept of critical colonization as a bacterial aided state of delayed healing without all the clinical signs of infection.

Dr Stephen Thomas *et al* reassess the role of maggot therapy in chronic wounds. He clarifies the appropriate wound characteristics and the cost effectiveness of applying large numbers of maggots for a short period of time. This therapy has its proponents and detractors but we are in need of defining and further studying the appropriate use of this therapy, especially properly controlled comparative studies with other debridement methods

The fourth chapter, by Rachael Walsh, explores the earlier diagnosis of malignant leg ulcers through community nurses performing skin biopsies and reducing the number of referrals to medical specialists or hospital clinics. Unnecessary visits could be eliminated with an earlier diagnosis and appropriate specific treatment to remove the malignancy.

Linda Russell facilitates the comparison and contrasting of various pressure ulcer classification systems helping us to identify common pitfalls in all the systems. These classification systems are only useful if continuous education is targeted at the clinician and I agree with her plea for national (and even international) consensus.

Lymphoedema is discussed by Jane Board and Wendy Harlow, taking the reader from an understanding of the components of the lymphatic system to a classification of the signs, symptoms and diagnosis. Lymphoedema is chronic, debilitating and often progressive, taxing the clinician's diagnostic and therapeutic skills. This well organized primer will help clinicians to assess accurately and communicate to patients the pathogenesis of lymphoedema and facilitate an appreciation of the treatment strategies.

In *Chapter 7*, Jacqueline Reilly takes us from an epidemiological study of 2202 surgical patients to a mathematical model of wound infection and surveillance. She distils the clinical application by informing us that the incidence of post operative infections is lower if the dressings are non-adherent and suture material is removed before ten days postoperatively.

Wound debridement, as discussed by O'Brien, is essential to remove dead or devitalized tissue, especially in those wounds with the ability to heal. The practitioner has several options for removing dead tissue, but we must be familiar with the risks and benefits of each modality and our clinical expertise before selecting the method for each wound. Sharp debridement training must be followed by a period of mentorship or preceptorship before competence can be translated into effective performance.

Are you currently using antiseptics in your practice? Do they have a role in the control of antibiotic resistant bacteria? The answers are not black and white but in this chapter, Scanlon and Stubbs examine the benefits, risks and costs to help integrate these agents into the appropriate management of complex wounds.

In the last chapter, Springett and White, define the skin changes of the foot at risk. The recognition of early warning signs and a prevention programme can help to save limbs.

This book will facilitate the continuing professional development of every wound care provider, as well as to stimulate the consideration of new and evolving paradigms in wound care. It is all too easy to let everyday practice become routine unless we open our minds to new perspectives and expand our clinical skills by examining our patients with new eyes.

Gary Sibbald MD
Associate Professor of Medicine
Director of Continuing Education
Department of Medicine
Director of Wound Healing Clinic, Sunnybrook and Women's College
University of Toronto

Chairperson, Education Committee
World Union of Wound Healing Societies

1

The wound healing continuum

David Gray, Richard J White, Pam Cooper

Wound classification systems have been devised in an attempt to provide simple frameworks for non-specialist nurses to assess and manage wounds. However, most have been seen to fail, probably due to over-simplification and failure to validate their usefulness. We have devised a classification system of healing that is based on colour and is an extrapolation of some of those that have gone before. We have taken the time to address the needs of the less experienced carer and have a more inclusive scheme. This is intended to aid identification of the main prognostic feature of the wound, which will serve as an indicator for healing or non-healing and provide the basis for selection of treatment. When used in conjunction with the wound infection continuum, we believe this system will provide an accurate framework sufficient to guide classification and management of most acute and chronic wounds.

Historically, there have been numerous wound classification systems, some broad-based and general, others specific to a particular wound type. None has received universal acclaim and all have been criticized for shortcomings, whether actual or perceived. All, however, have been intended to aid management of the patient — from the simplistic systems intended for basic education, through to the esoteric and highly technical systems intended for the expert.

Some classification systems have depended on a simple colour coding (Cuzzell, 1988; Stotts, 1990; Krasner, 1995; Lorentzen *et al*, 1999). Each of these has relied on a spectrum of colours — red, yellow and black — to equate with granulation, slough and necrosis respectively. By estimating the proportions of each colour present in any given wound, one can use this as an adjunct to traditional classification according to aetiology, dimensions, bacterial contamination and so on. It has been claimed that this colour system helps identify which phase of the healing continuum a wound is in, and, as a consequence, broad guidelines on management. For example, a yellow 'sloughy' wound requires debridement (Krasner, 1995). However, even the author admitted the shortcomings of this generalization by describing two types of yellow wound — the sloughy and the infected/pus-filled. Red can also be too broad a descriptor; granulating, healthy wounds are red as are wounds colonized or infected with haemolytic streptococci. Following a few years of use, the simple, three-colour system has largely fallen into disuse even though a 'moderate' inter-observer correlation has been reported (Lorentzen *et al*, 1999). The three-colour system has been labelled 'an over-simplification' (Hilton and Harding, 2001).

Kingsley (2001) has devised a wound infection continuum. This, too, is a framework for clinical practice. It relies on an understanding of some commonly-used terms and a spectrum which extends from the sterile to the infected wound. This continuum has been further clarified (White *et al*, 2002) and is the basis of *Chapter 2* (White, 2002).

The wound healing continuum (WHC) that we have devised relies on the identification of the colours present in any given wound and applying the most clinically significant to the spectrum, which extends from black to pink with intermediate gradations (*Figure 1.1*). This system is not intended to replace any of those already extant, rather, it is a supplemental and general system. The overriding principle which dictates the most clinically significant colour is the need to address that component to permit wound healing. So, in a wound that contains any black eschar, the primary requirement is to debride before healing can proceed — without this intervention, there will be no healing. This is illustrated in *Figure 1.2*.

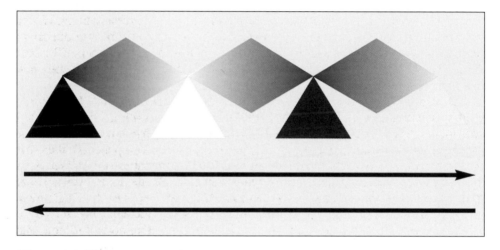

Figure 1.1: The wound healing continuum

The development of the WHC does allow the majority of wounds that heal by secondary intention to be included. There will always be exceptions. One of the problems we have with any classification — be it of pressure ulcers or risk assessment, etc. — is that people have failed to recognize the anomalies and limitations at the very start.

The two user-friendly continuums discussed in this book can guide clinical decision-making for basic staff, or staff who do not work with wounds on a regular basis.

The basis of identification

Which colour is of primary importance? As the continuum is followed from left to right, ie. from black to pink, it correlates with healing of the wound. Not all wounds will naturally progress in this fashion. Not all wounds will exhibit black. In general, it is most important to identify the colour that is furthest to the left of the continuum, then to implement management procedures to eradicate that colour, enabling the wound to progress steadily to the right. Again, generally speaking, each colour or combination will dictate a specific wound management approach. There are exceptions to this rule, but our aim is to use the WHC to support clinical decision making, not to replace it. This chapter does not address the management methodology.

The black wound

Black has been termed the 'unhealthiest' colour (Stotts, 1990). It is typical of necrosis and has connotations of gangrene and of malignant melanoma. However, black does not always have serious repercussions, as not all black wounds are gangrenous. The fully black wound, covered by dry, hard eschar is illustrated in *Figure 1.2*. This is a typical, benign presentation of the heel pressure ulcer. Where the wound under consideration is a pressure ulcer, it might also be appropriate to refer to a specific classification system at all stages of management (Russell, 2002). Such a classification will include wound characteristics such as depth, and risk factors associated with the individual patient.

Clearly, in this instance debridement is essential (Torrance, 1983). The method used will be dictated by local policy, formulary and the skills of the individual practitioner. Not all heels will present fully covered with eschar, however, where the ulcer is 'multicoloured' (ie. has red, yellow and other components) then the principle is to classify according to the black. For a wound that has progressed from this early stage, using the same heel wound as an example, the initial debridement of eschar often reveals yellow slough beneath. This then becomes the single most important feature to classify. It dictates that further debridement, possibly by a different approach to that taken previously, is required. It is important to note that the presence of black tissue in a wound is not restricted to pressure ulcers. Acute wounds, such as surgical wounds, will occasionally develop hard, dry eschar.

The black-yellow wound

This wound should be classified as a black wound as this is the more 'serious' colour on the continuum. The yellow component usually indicates the presence of fibrous slough, which frequently co-exists with eschar (*Figure 1.3*). A wound presenting with these two colours may be deteriorating to the left of the continuum, or improving as eschar is removed. Consequently, the past history of the progress of the wound, and of the patient's general condition, must be ascertained.

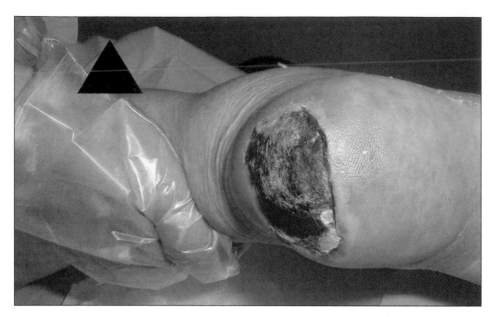

Figure 1.2: The black wound

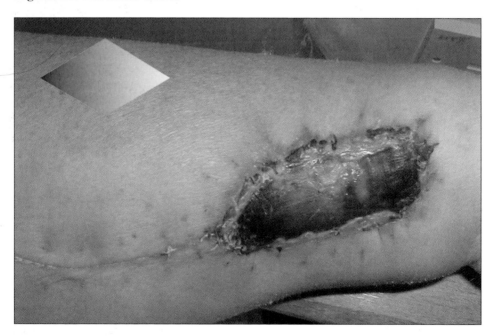

Figure 1.3: The black-yellow wound

The yellow wound

For any wound with a yellow component, first consider the possibility of pus and therefore infection. Once this has been eliminated as a possible reason, then yellow is attributable to slough (Tong, 1999) (*Figure 1.4*). Slough is usually yellow but may also be white; it serves as a medium for the growth of bacteria and must, therefore, be removed (Tong, 1999).

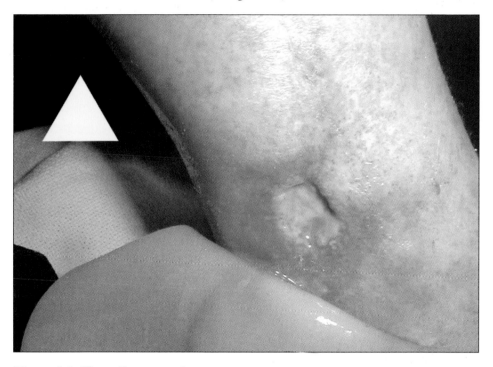

Figure 1.4: The yellow wound

The yellow-red wound

As with all bicoloured or multicoloured wounds (*Figure 1.5*), the wound should be classified according to the most serious colour. In this case the red component is probably due to granulation tissue. However, not all red is positive — some may be attributable to colonization or infection with a haemolytic bacterium such as β-haemolytic *Streptococcus* species (groups A, B, C and G; Schraibman, 1990). These organisms are well-known pathogens in leg ulcers and burns/plastic surgery. Red may also be attributable to the presence of frank blood, possibly from friable granulation tissue (an infection criterion), or trauma. Once these factors have been eliminated as causes, then granulation tissue remains as the most likely explanation.

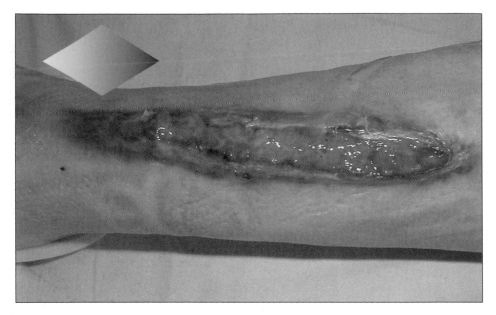

Figure 1.5: The yellow-red wound

The red wound

As stated in the red/yellow section, not all red tissue may be healthy or beneficial to the patient. However, once all other potential causes of the red tissue are excluded it would be reasonable to assume that the wound is filled with healthy granulation tissue (*Figure 1.6*). It should be remembered that the red tissue may develop unhealthy characteristics such as critical colonization (Kingsley, 2001) and consideration should be given to this fact. Critical colonization of previously healthy granular tissue will result in it failing to heal and possible deterioration in the wound bed.

The red-pink wound

In *Figure 1.7* the wound can be seen to have virtually covered the granulation tissue with fresh epithelium. At this stage the wound requires a stable, moist environment to ensure the epithelialization process can be completed.

The pink 'wound'

This is not a wound as such — the pink is due to the growth of new epithelium and so the wound has healed (*Figure 1.8*). It may, however, still require protection until the tissues have consolidated.

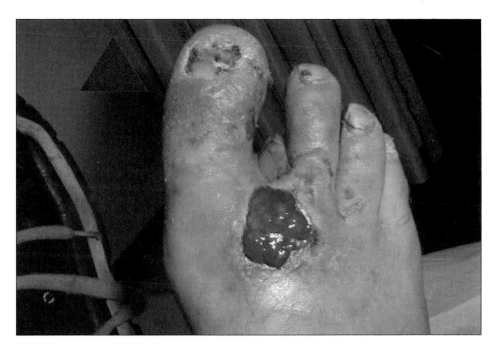

Figure 1.6: The red wound

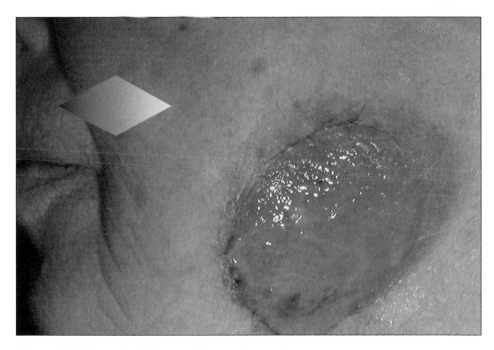

Figure 1.7: The red-pink wound

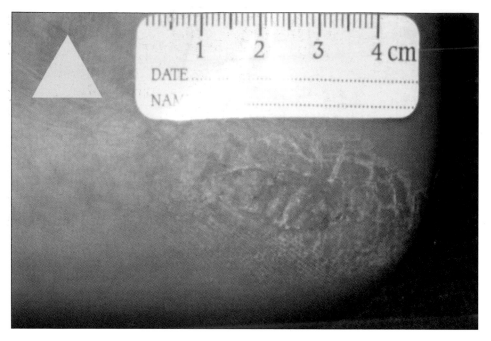

Figure 1.8: The pink wound

Infected wounds

Wounds that are showing signs of green or blue (*Figure 1.9*) are almost certainly colonized or critically colonized with bacteria (Kingsley, 2001). Typically the bacterium *Pseudomonas aeruginosa* will provide a green/blue colour to the wound (Villavicencio, 1998). In such cases, control of bioburden will be required (White *et al*, 2002). This will be dependant on many factors, eg. the patient's intercurrent illnesses, concomitant medications, risk factors, etc. These wounds are not included within the WHC as they need to be assessed using the wound infection continuum. Using both continuums provides maximum support to the user.

Multiple colour wounds

Many wounds will present with a variety of different coloured tissue. As seen in *Figure 1.10* this wound presents with every colour from the WHC. However, by focusing management on the removal of the tissue with the colour closest to the left-hand side of the continuum — in this case black tissue – the wound can be moved along the continuum towards the right/pink end point. As seen in *Figure 1.11*, within seven days the wound has moved to the yellow/red category. In effect, by focusing management on the tissue colour closest to the left-hand side of the continuum, the wound has in seven days been moved in a positive fashion towards healing.

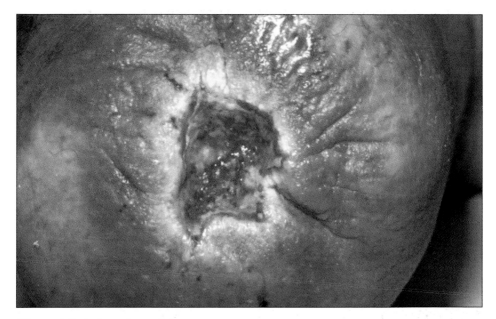

Figure 1.9: Infected wound

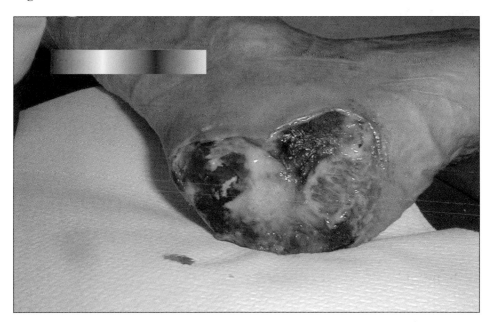

Figure 1.10: The rainbow wound

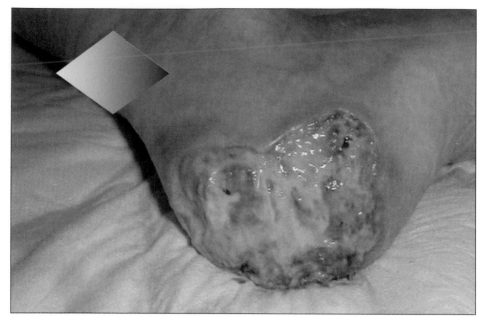

Figure 1.11: The rainbow wound has become a yellow-red wound

Discussion

At present, little or nothing is known of healing rates in relation to open wounds healing by secondary intention in the UK. To remedy this lack of information clinical audits are required, which consider the time taken to heal wounds such as pressure ulcers on the heel. Such clinical audits would require a classification tool which would allow for the inclusion of most wounds healing by secondary intention. It is our belief that audits currently under way using the WHC may identify it as a classification tool suitable for such use. Only when baseline audit data is in place will practitioners be able to assess their own healing rates and effectively reflect on their practice. Further work is required to identify the strengths and weaknesses of the WHC. Once such work has been completed, it may be that the WHC and the wound infection continuum will be seen as effective aids to clinical practice in the field of wound healing.

Conclusions

Within this chapter, the authors have sought to introduce a new continuum which can assist in the categorization of most wounds healing by secondary intention. When used in conjunction with the wound infection continuum, the user can receive guidance as to the condition of the wound. Both continuums, if used correctly, could also aid long term clinical audit.

Key points

⌘ Classification systems are a useful tool in aiding clinical decision making.

⌘ Existing wound healing classifications have been criticized for being overly simplistic.

⌘ The wound healing continuum proposed here relies on the identification of the colours present in any given wound and applying the most clinically significant to the spectrum, which extends from black to pink with intermediate gradations.

⌘ When used in conjunction with the wound infection continuum, the wound healing continuum forms a useful basis for assessment, classification and management of wounds.

References

Cuzzell JZ (1988) The new red, yellow, black color code. *Am J Nurs* **88**(10): 1342–46

Hilton J, Harding KG (2001) Wound bed preparation: a physician's clinical experience. In: Cherry GW, Harding KG, Ryan TJ, eds. *Wound Bed Preparation*. The Royal Society of Medicine Press, London

Kingsley A (2001) A proactive approach to wound infection. *Nurs Standard* **11**(15): 50–8

Krasner D (1995) Wound care: how to use the red-yellow-black system. *Am J Nurs* **95**(5): 44–7

Lorentzen HF, Holstein P, Gottrup F (1999) Interobservatorvariation ved rodt-gult-sort-sarbeskrivelsessystemet. *Ugeskr Laeger* **161**(44): 6045–8

Russell L (2002) Pressure ulcer classification: the systems and the pitfalls. *Br J Nurs* **11**(12 Suppl): 49–59

Schraibman IG (1990) The significance of β-haemolytic streptococci in chronic leg ulcers. *Ann R Coll Surg Engl* **72**: 123–4

Stotts NA (1990) Seeing red and yellow and black. The three-color concept of wound care. *Nursing* **20**(2): 59–61

Tong A (1999) The identification and treatment of slough. *J Wound Care* **8**(7): 338–9

Torrance C (1983) *Pressure Sores. Aetiology, Treatment and Prevention*. Croom Helm, London and Canberra

Villavicencio RT (1998) The history of blue pus. *J Am Coll Surg* **187**(2): 212–16

White RJ (2002) The wound infection continuum. *Br J Nurs* **11**(22 Suppl): 7–9

White RJ, Cooper R, Kingsley A (2002) A topical issue: the use of antibacterials in wound pathogen control. In: White RJ, ed. *Trends in Wound Care*. Quay Books, MA Healthcare Limited, Salisbury

2

The wound infection continuum

Richard J White

For many people, a wound is either 'infected' or 'not infected'. However, this binary distinction is too simplistic: between these descriptions is a spectrum of microbial involvement. This spectrum has been termed the 'infection continuum', and is a framework for classification, assessment and management of the wound and its microbial load (or bioburden). By recognition of pre-infected stages and appropriate intervention, the progression of a wound to infection could be avoided. Such avoidance would benefit the patient and, by lowering costs, the healthcare system.

Although most wounds heal without difficulty, some will become infected and cause increased morbidity such as pain and loss of function. In some cases, wound infection leads to mortality and, in all cases, increased intensity of healthcare intervention with inpatient stay increases costs. Prevention of infection is therefore desirable.

The transition from acute healing wound to chronic non-healing wound can be avoided by prompt intervention to stop infection (White *et al*, 2001, 2002). This intervention is based on microbiological concepts, knowledge of the normal healing process, and correct interpretation of clinical signs in the wound and the patient.

Heavy microbial load (bioburden) in the wound is probably the most important and common factor in a disordered healing process (Halbert *et al*, 1992; Cooper and Lawrence, 1996a,b; Bowler *et al*, 2001). Delayed healing is the result of disordered cellular cascades stimulated by an unbalanced wound microbe population, causing cellular dysfunction and subsequent biochemical imbalance. Once dysfunction and imbalance are established, they can be resistant to adjustment with commonly used wound-care interventions, as well as being a challenge to more costly emerging therapies, such as protease inhibitors, growth factors and extracellular matrix components (Bowler, 2002). These clinical problems may be addressed by the practice of 'wound bed preparation' and the use of specific protease-modulating treatments (Sibbald *et al*, 2000; Cullen *et al*, 2002; Ghatnekar *et al*, 2002; Vin *et al*, 2002; Veves *et al*, 2002). The presence and implications of microorganisms in the wound have recently been described in terms of a continuum: this provides the framework for the assessment and management of wound bioburden (Dow *et al*, 1999; Kingsley, 2001).

The infection continuum is a framework for the assessment and diagnosis of wounds that are colonized or infected, and is best used in conjunction with the wound healing continuum (*Chapter 1*; [Gray *et al*, 2002]).

Diagnosis of wound infection

Clinical features

Several signs and symptoms accompany wound infection, but not all wounds will exhibit these at any one time. However, there are 'cardinal' or 'classic' signs that are characteristic in every case: for example, spreading erythema or frank pus. In many cases, the presentation is more complex or subtle. Although erythema around an acute wound in healthy skin, or pus in an otherwise clean wound, would be clearly evident, the same signs in a sloughy leg ulcer with varicose eczema and lipodermatosclerosis would be harder to recognize. To distinguish acute and chronic wounds for the purposes of infection criteria is therefore advisable. The current standard infection criteria are those of Cutting and Harding (1994) (*Table 2.1*). They have been validated by Gardner *et al* (2001), who found increasing pain and wound breakdown to be the most sensitive indicators of wound infection.

Table 2.1: Criteria for wound infection
Abscess
Cellulitis
Discharge
Delayed healing
Discolouration
Friable, bleeding granulation tissue
Unexpected pain/tenderness
Pocketing/bridging at base of the wound
Abnormal smell
Wound breakdown

Source: Cutting and Harding, 1994

Systemic signs of infection such as raised white cell count (neutropenia) and raised serum C-reactive protein (CRP) are standard blood measurements for infection. However, for chronic infected wounds such as leg ulcers, raised CRP may not be diagnostic (Goodfield, 1988).

Microbiological features

During World War I, clinicians recognized that wounds with high microbial loads (or low concentrations of β-haemolytic streptococci) were prone to infection and best healed by secondary intention. The relation between raised microbial numbers and wound infection has been reinforced by several studies (Bornside and Bornside, 1979) and 10^5 cfu/g or 10^5 cfu/cm^2 became accepted as the thresholds that normally indicate infection when exceeded. ('Cfu' denotes 'colony-forming units', which are single microbial cells or clumps of cells that form distinct colonies when grown *in vitro*: a representation of viable counting in microbiology.) The 10^5 threshold has been critically examined by Bowler (2003) who concluded that treatment should be based on achieving a host-manageable bioburden rather than relying on a quantitative criterion.

Robson (1997) has discussed the need to maintain a balance in bacterial numbers to promote unimpeded healing. He has concluded that at densities of less than 10^5 cfu/g, granulation tissue formation proceeds, whereas at higher densities it does not. However, the presence of β-haemolytic streptococci, even at low concentrations, is capable of impeding healing (Schraibman, 1990). Since quantitative analysis is not done in the UK, these criteria are not easily applied.

'Diagnosis' or recognition of critical colonization

The quantity and diversity of microbes (bioburden) representing colonization, critical colonization and infection are individual and depend on the quality of immune response of the host to tackle the particular mix of microbes present. They are not, therefore, exact states; nor are they easily definable by microbiological characterization or quantification, but are likely to follow in order from left to right on the continuum (*Figure 2.1*).

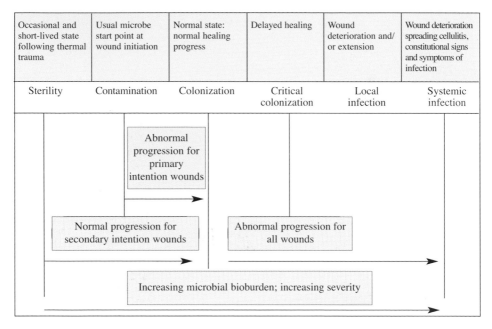

Figure 2.1: The wound infection continuum (adapted from Kingsley, 2001)

Some wounds progress quickly from colonization to infection via a clinically indistinct critical colonization state. Such wounds change suddenly and noticeably from normal healing to abnormal deterioration, without ever stopping at a mid-point of 'indolence' or delayed healing. Others will move from colonization to the abnormal critical state and remain there as an indolent, but not visibly deteriorating, wound.

This movement is likely to occur for two reasons (*Figure 2.2*). First, although initially weighted heavily in favour of wound healing due to the host immunocompetency from good health and/or control of underlying diseases, the balance will change in the opposing direction if immunocompetency falls. The existing wound bioburden can now exceed its usual level. The host's controlling immune response can no longer cope with the microbial load. Second, the bioburden increases in quantity or is joined by newly cross-contaminating microbes that increase the virulence of the mixture present, outweighing the immunocompetency on the other end of the scales. When the scales balance, the states of colonization and critical colonization exist, and strategies such as the use of antiseptics to reduce the 'weight' (the total number and/or number of species present) of the bioburden will tip the scales back towards healing (Fumal *et al*, 2002). In essence, good wound care adds weight to the right-hand side of the scales. The governing factor in wound infection is the immune response, ie. the host response. Appropriate use of topical antimicrobials can work with the host response to control bioburden and restore healing.

The situation in which the balance is tipped towards infection may coincide either with the expression of virulence factors by the pathogens or with a reduction in the quality of the host response (*Figure 2.2*). There is no evidence to support one factor over the other (Heinzelmann *et al*, 2002).

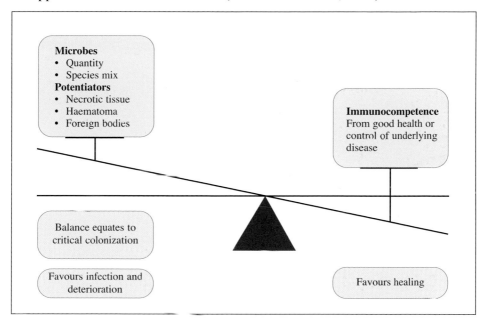

Figure 2.2: The balance of factors influencing possible wound infection

This state of critical colonization is most likely to equate biochemically and in cellular terms with the late inflammation phase of the wound healing process.

Clinical appearance of critical colonization

❖ Indolent wound, not responding to appropriate care of wound (topical dressings) and underlying pathologies (eg. removal of pressure, reversal of venous hypertension), with no cellulitis.

❖ Exacerbation of pain, or pain becomes present when it was not before, or change in the quality/experience of pain, still without manifest cellulitis.

❖ Thick slough not responding to standard techniques (eg. hydrogels, hydrocolloids).

❖ Fast-returning slough after rapid debridement techniques (eg. larval, sharp/surgical).
❖ Intransigent odour.

Conclusions

The wound-infection continuum is a framework for the assessment of wounds according to microbiological influences. It assists in the identification of key stages of host-pathogen interaction, and so helps in the decision-making leading to antimicrobial therapy. The concept of critical colonization is central to the continuum. It is useful in understanding the role of pathogens in delayed healing and, consequently, can also determine treatment.

When used in conjunction with the healing continuum, this framework for clinical practice can provide the basis for the assessment and classification of most wounds. Further studies are needed to confirm the clinical usefulness of this approach.

Key points

⌘ Diagnosis of infection is based on signs and symptoms in the first instance.

⌘ Microbiological investigations can be useful in identifying pathogens and their antimicrobial sensitivity, and in interpreting clinical data.

⌘ Awareness of the concept of critical colonization is useful in explaining some cases of delayed healing.

⌘ When used in conjunction with the wound-healing continuum, the wound infection continuum forms a useful basis for assessment, classification and management of wounds.

⌘ Treatment interventions should be based on the need to achieve a host manageable bioburden. Intervention at an early stage, eg. critical colonization, can avoid progression to infection and increased morbidity.

References

Bornside GH, Bornside BB (1979) Comparison between moist swab and tissue biopsy methods for bacteria in experimental incision wounds. *J Trauma* **19**: 103–5

Bowler PG, Duerden BI, Armstrong DG (2001) Wound microbiology and associated approaches to wound management. *Clin Microbiol Rev* **14**(2): 244–69

Bowler PG (2002) Wound pathophysiology, infection and therapeutic options. *Ann Med* **34**: 419–27

Bowler PG (2003) The 10^5 bacterial growth guideline: reassessing its clinical relevance in wound healing. *Ostomy, Management* **49**(1): 44–53

Cooper R, Lawrence JC (1996a) Micro-organisms and wounds. *J Wound Care* **5**(5): 233–6

Cooper R, Lawrence JC (1996b) The prevalence of bacteria and implications for infection control. *J Wound Care* **5**(6): 291–5

Cullen B, Smith R, McCulloch E, Silcock D, Morrison L (2002) Mechanism of action of Promogran, a protease modulating matrix, for the treatment of diabetic foot ulcers. *J Wound Repair Regen* **10**(1): 16–25

Cutting KF, Harding KG (1994) Criteria for identifying wound infection. *J Wound Care* **3**(4): 198–201

Dow G, Browne A, Sibbald G (1999) Infection in chronic wounds. Controversies in diagnosis and treatment. *Ostomy, Wound Management* **45**(8): 23–40

Fumal I, Braham C, Paquet P, Pierard-Franchimont C, Pierard GE (2002) The beneficial toxicity paradox of antimicrobials in leg ulcer healing impaired by a polymicrobial flora: a proof of concept study. *Dermatology* **204**(Suppl 1): 70–4

Gardner S *et al* (2001) The validity of the clinical signs and symptoms used to identify localised wound infection. *Wound Repair Regen* **9**(3): 178–86

Ghatnekar O, Willis M, Persson U (2002) Cost-effectiveness of treating deep diabetic foot ulcers with Promogran in four European countries. *J Wound Care* **11**(2): 70–4

Goodfield MJ (1988) C-reactive protein levels in venous ulceration: an indication of infection? *J Am Acad Dermatol* **18**(5): 1048–52

Gray D, White RJ, Cooper P (2002) The wound healing continuum. *Br J Nurs* **11**(22 suppl): 15–19

Halbert AR, Stacey MC, Rohr JB, Jopp-McKay A (1992) The effect of bacterial colonization on venous ulcer healing. *Aust J Dermatol* **33**: 75–80

Heinzelmann M, Scott M, Lan T (2002) Factors predisposing to bacterial invasion and infection. *Am J Surg* **183**: 179–90

Kingsley A (2001) A proactive approach to wound infection. *Nurs Standard* **15**(30): 50–8

Robson MC (1997) Wound infection: a failure of wound healing caused by an imbalance of bacteria. *Surg Clin North Am* **77**(3): 637–50

Schraibman IG (1990) The significance of β-haemolytic streptococci in chronic leg ulcers. *Ann Roy Coll Surg Eng* **72**: 123–4

Sibbald G, Williamson D, Orstcd HL, Campbell K, Keast D, Krasner D, Sibbald D (2000) Preparing the wound bed — debridement, bacterial balance, and moisture balance. *Ostomy, Wound Management* **46**(11): 14–35

Veves A, Sheehan P, Pham HT (2002) A randomized, controlled trial of Promogran (a collagen/oxidized regenerated cellulose dressing) vs standard treatment in the management of diabetic foot ulcers. *J Arch Surg* **137**(7): 822–7

Vin F, Teot L, Meaume S (2002) The healing properties of Promogran in venous leg ulcers. *J Wound Care* **11**(9): 335–41

White RJ, Cooper R, Kingsley A (2001) Wound colonization and infection: the role of topical antimicrobials. *Br J Nurs* **10**(9): 563–78

White R, Cooper RA, Kingsley A (2002) A topical issue: the use of antibacterials in wound pathogen control. In: White R, ed. *Trends in Wound Care*. Quay Books, MA Healthcare Limited, Dinton, Wiltshire: 16–36

3

The current status of maggot therapy in wound healing

Stephen Thomas, Mary Jones, Karen Wynn, Tony Fowler

The clinical use of sterile maggots under the brand name LarvE has increased steadily in the UK since they were introduced in the UK in late 1995. Some fifty articles have been published in the last four years that describe the cost-effectiveness of maggot therapy in a variety of wound types including leg ulcers, pressure ulcers and diabetic ulcers. The ability of these creatures to combat wound infection has been well documented, including those caused by antibiotic-resistant strains of bacteria such as methicillin-resistant Staphylococcus aureus. No significant risks or adverse events have been linked to the use of maggots, although their presence may increase pain levels in leg ulcers associated with ischaemic disease.

The popular practice in the twentieth century of introducing live maggots into wounds to carry out debridement or combat infection fell into decline with the introduction of antibiotics in the 1940s. It remained a scientific curiosity until the late 1980s when Dr Sherman, from the University of California, began to re-evaluate the technique for the treatment of pressure ulcers and other chronic wounds (Sherman *et al*, 1993).

Maggot therapy was reintroduced in the UK in late 1995, when sterile maggots of the common greenbottle *Lucilia sericata* were first produced under the brand name of LarvE by the Biosurgical Research Unit (BRU), an NHS laboratory based in the Princess of Wales Hospital, Bridgend. This chapter describes the current status of maggot therapy and discusses possible future developments.

Current status of maggot therapy

Since 1995, the BRU has supplied approximately 35000 vials of LarvE, containing about ten million maggots, to some 1300 centres throughout the UK and, despite the practical problems associated with the transportation of these live insects, to many European countries and as far as South Africa.

As a result of the clinical successes reported with LarvE, a number of production facilities have been established elsewhere throughout Europe, including Germany, Hungary, Sweden, Belgium, and the Ukraine, although details of the numbers of patients that have been treated by each centre are not available.

In 1996, the BRU organized the first international conference on biosurgery, following which the International Biotherapy Society was founded 'to investigate and develop the use of living organisms, or their products, in tissue repair'. A series of further successful international conferences on maggot therapy has been held in South Wales, Israel, and Germany, the latest being held in Turkey in May 2003.

Clinical evidence

Over sixty articles have been published in the last six years that describe the use of maggots. While some are reviews or digests of previously published articles (Sherman, 1998; Thomas, 1998) others contain the results of clinical assessments or consist of illustrated case reports that describe the use of maggots in a variety of wound types including pressure ulcers (Sherman *et al*, 1995b; Thomas *et al*, 1996a,b), leg ulcers (Thomas 1996a,b), diabetic foot wounds (Evans, 1997; Mumcuoglu *et al*, 1997; Rayman *et al*, 1998), traumatic wounds (Thomas *et al*, 1996a), various types of surgical wounds (Gacheru, 1998; Jones and Champion, 1998), burns (Namias *et al*, 2000), and an infected insect bite (Chaffrey, 1997).

In addition to these largely anecdotal reports, three studies have been published in which some element of control has been attempted. Two involve small groups of patients with pressure ulcers (Sherman *et al*, 1993) and leg ulcers (Wayman *et al*, 2000, 2001) and, in the third (Stoddard *et al*, 1995), a patient with bilateral ulcers acted as his own control.

The authors of one of these investigations (Wayman *et al*, 2000, 2001) also produced data on the cost-effectiveness of LarvE treatment compared with that of a conventional dressing designed to promote autolytic wound debridement. In this twelve-patient study, the average expenditure on materials to debride successfully one leg ulcer was £69.53 with maggots and £319.56 with hydrogel. The debriding rates achieved for wounds dressed with hydrogel was 2/6 in one month, (33%) and are comparable with those of earlier clinical trials involving hydrogel dressings, which ranged from 21% in twenty-one days to 38% in twenty-eight days (Thomas and Jones, 2001).

Preliminary results of a large randomized controlled trial involving 140 patients with diabetic foot wounds were presented to the Biosurgical Conference in Bridgend in 2001 (Turner, 2001). This study, which was undertaken by a multidisciplinary team in Lviv Medical University, Ukraine, also showed similar dramatic differences in debridement rates for these two treatments. These publications support the observations made over sixty years ago that maggots promote rapid debridement, combat infection and promote healing.

Key practical aspects of maggot therapy

The number of maggots required to achieve rapid debridement is determined principally by the size of the wound and the amount of necrotic tissue present. Originally, a maximum of about ten maggots per cm^2 was recommended (Robinson, 1934), but now it is recognized that provided the surrounding skin is protected using an appropriate dressing technique (Thomas *et al*, 1998; Thomas and Jones, 1999), the maximum number of maggots used is probably not critical.

A simple calculator (*Figure 3.1*), available from the BRU, can be used to provide basic guidance on the number of pots required (there are about 300 maggots per pot) for different sized wounds containing varying amounts of slough or necrotic tissue. Clinical experience has shown that, in the long term, it is much more cost-effective to use a small number of treatments involving large numbers of maggots than extended treatments with small numbers of maggots.

LarvE® Calculator

The *LarvE*® Calculator indicates the recommended number of pots of sterile maggots required per application to achieve rapid debridement of sloughy/infected wounds.

Maximum wound size (cm)	Percentage of wound area covered with slough				
	20%	40%	60%	80%	100%
Up to 2 x 2					
5 x 5					
5 x 10					
10 x 10					
10 x 15					
15 x 15					
15 x 20					
20 x 20					
20 x 25					
25 x 25					
30 x 30					

© SMTL 2000

Number of pots

0.5		1		2		3		4		5	

Measure the dimensions of the wound and compare with the wound sizes indicated on the side of the calculator. Move horizontally across the table to the column that most likely corresponds to the percentage of the wound area covered with slough. The number of pots required is indicated by the colour shown.

For advice on the number of pots for the treatment of specific wounds please contact the Biosurgical Research Unit on 01656 752820.

Although these recommendations are based on extensive clinical experience with the technique, the final decision on the number of pots to be applied must remain the responsibility of the practitioner providing the treatment.

Figure 3.1: LarvE calculator

Maggot enzymes appear to function optimally at around pH 8–8.5. In an acidic environment the ability of these enzymes to function normally may be impaired. It follows, therefore, that in wounds that have a marked acidic pH as a result of their metabolic activity, the ability of small, newly hatched maggots to survive and develop normally may be compromised.

It is interesting to speculate if the pretreatment of such a wound with an appropriate buffer or a rinse with a solution of sodium bicarbonate might change the wound pH sufficiently to allow the maggots to become established. To the best of our knowledge this approach has not been tried clinically. Even under ideal conditions a small proportion of maggots applied to the wound may not survive. There is, therefore, no point in counting the number of maggots applied and attempting to reconcile this figure with the number of full grown maggots present at the end of the treatment.

When using maggots it is important to ensure that any secondary dressings permit the ingress of oxygen and the free drainage of excess wound fluid. Semipermeable film dressings should not be used. Research has shown that although maggot development is unaffected either by therapeutic doses of several commonly used antibiotics (Sherman *et al*, 1995a) or exposure to high doses of X-rays (Surgical Materials Testing Laboratory [SMTL], unpublished data), their development can be adversely affected by the presence within the wound of residues of hydrogel dressings containing propylene glycol (Thomas and Andrews, 1999). All traces of such gels should, therefore, be removed from the wound before the application of LarvE.

Mode of action

As they move around within a wound, maggots produce secretions containing proteolytic enzymes that break down necrotic tissue into a semiliquid form that they subsequently ingest — the basis of their wound cleansing action.

The ability of maggots to combat wound infection, including that caused by antibiotic-resistant strains of bacteria, such as methicillin-resistant *Staphylococcus aureus*, is the result of at least two mechanisms:

1. The antimicrobial activity of their external secretions (Freidman *et al*, 1998; Thomas *et al*, 1999).
2. The destruction within the insects' gut of viable organisms that are taken up during their normal feeding activity (Mumcuoglu *et al*, 2001).

Maggot secretions have also been shown in laboratory studies to accelerate the growth of mammalian fibroblast cells in culture (Prete, 1997). This stimulatory activity may explain the reported ability of maggots to accelerate the healing of some chronic wounds. In particular, with difficult or long-standing chronic wounds, there may be some benefit in applying maggots after the initial cleansing stage has been completed to prevent reinfection and stimulate the healing process; however, further work is required to confirm this hypothesis.

Contraindications and adverse reactions to maggot therapy

A review of the literature reveals no significant risks or adverse events related to the clinical use of sterile maggots, although larval enzymes can cause significant excoriation if they are allowed to run on to unprotected skin around the margin of a wound. This problem may be overcome by protecting the surrounding skin before the application of the maggots. In severe cases, this results in superficial skin damage, which rapidly resolves within a few days (Thomas *et al*, 1996b).

The most common problem with maggot therapy is that of physical discomfort. This can vary from a mild 'picking' sensation to pain that is so severe that it leads to premature termination of the treatment. Experience with the technique in the UK suggests that such pain is most commonly associated with the use of maggots in the treatment of ischaemic limbs. It has also been noted that the pain is generally eliminated immediately after the maggots are removed from the wound and it is postulated that the pain is the result of an increase in wound pH known to result from the metabolic activity of the maggots.

If wound-related pain becomes a serious problem the use of potent analgesics should be considered. Generally, however, and perhaps surprisingly, patient acceptance of the technique has been very high (Sherman, 1998).

A transient pyrexia has been reported in some patients, as described previously (McLellan, 1932), but its aetiology has never been satisfactorily explained. It is possible that this might be the result of the absorption of pyrogenic material that is released from the cell walls of Gram-negative bacteria that are lysed during their passage through the maggots' gut.

Importance of education, training and technical support

Although maggot therapy is not difficult to perform, as with any clinical procedure, effective training is key to a successful outcome. The BRU offers regular practical training sessions in Bridgend, where healthcare professionals can update their knowledge of larval therapy. Similar training days can also be organized at other locations around the country by arrangement with the BRU.

As part of the ongoing educational process, a website for LarvE has been established (http://www.Larvae.com).

Future of maggot therapy

The long-term future of maggot therapy will depend upon a number of factors. Although many clinicians have seen for themselves the benefits of maggot therapy and are therefore happy to use it for a wide range of clinical conditions, others remain unconvinced, citing the absence of well-controlled clinical studies to support its more widespread use.

This issue is likely to be addressed by the Health Technology Assessment Programme. This organization has published a request for interested parties to apply for funding to conduct meaningful studies on maggot therapy in accordance with the stringent criteria required for the results to be included in a systematic review. It is hoped that the eventual findings of these investigations will be sufficiently unambiguous to convince even the most skeptical clinicians of the value of maggot therapy.

A further barrier to the extended use of maggot therapy is its exclusion from the Drug Tariff, which seriously limits its availability in the community where the majority of wounds are to be found. A Drug Tariff listing would make maggots available to patients in the primary healthcare sector, which could result in a marked reduction in hospital admissions for wounds such as diabetic ulcers and other chronic lesions.

Numerous centres around the world are known to be actively engaged in isolating and characterizing some of the secretions produced by *Lucilia sericata* (confidential information). The intention is that these could then be synthesized and incorporated into a convenient topical pharmaceutical formulation in order to replace the live maggot as a therapeutic agent.

Although there is no theoretical reason why this should not be done, it is unlikely that the once-daily application of individual agents prepared in this way would be as clinically effective as the maggots themselves, as practical experience with other commercially available enzymatic debriding agents has proved disappointing. Maggots continuously produce a cocktail of bioactive agents within the wound while combating infection by digesting and killing living bacteria actively.

It is likely that other fly species known to cause benign myiasis of human wounds may produce mixtures of enzymes with subtle differences from those produced by *Lucilia sericata*. Currently, no information is available on the comparative efficacy of these different species in the clinical situation. Clearly this is an area that could form the subject of some interesting research.

In Germany, Dr W Fleischman has described how maggots enclosed in a soft polyvinylalcohol foam bag can be applied to wounds. The principal advantage of this system is claimed to be that the maggots are easier to apply and remove while remaining invisible both to the user and the patient. The disadvantages are that the maggots are not able to move around freely within the wound to focus upon areas of necrotic tissue or work their way into infected pockets or sinuses. The ability of the maggots to combat infection by ingesting bacteria may also be compromised and debridement times are also likely to be significantly increased. Nevertheless, the technique may offer certain advantages for flat wounds or those in the perineal area, and as such is actively being investigated by the BRU.

Conclusion

Since maggot therapy was reintroduced in 1995, it has grown rapidly in popularity although not all healthcare professionals have embraced the idea enthusiastically. Some hospitals use large numbers of maggots apparently to good effect, while similar hospitals elsewhere may use none at all. Similar differences exist between different departments in a single hospital or even between different consultants working in the same specialty in a single hospital.

In the light of the often dramatic results reported by many users of maggots, it is difficult to understand the reasons or justification for these differences. A personal prejudice against maggots on the part of the clinician (be it doctor or nurse) should not prevent a patient receiving a therapy, no matter how unusual, that might make a positive contribution to that individual's care, particularly in the case of patients for whom the only alternative is surgery or an unwanted amputation. Maggot therapy will not always work, but it is almost always worth considering save in the most extreme or unfavourable conditions.

It should always be remembered, however, that maggots cannot do the impossible. For example, it is pointless to apply them to a leg where the blood supply is totally inadequate to maintain tissue perfusion. To do so is to waste resources and delays the inevitable amputation. It is also unrealistic to expect a single application of maggots to do in three days what conventional treatments have failed to achieve in months. In such extreme cases, multiple applications with an adequate number of maggots may be required to bring about a significant improvement in the condition of a wound.

Key points

⌘   Maggot therapy which is no longer regarded as the treatment of last resort, is widely used throughout the UK for treatment of all types of infected/necrotic wounds.

⌘   Studies have shown that the cost of wound debridement with LarvE is less than that of conventional techniques.

⌘   It is more cost-effective to apply large numbers of maggots for a short period than to use insufficient numbers, which will result in extended treatment times. The new LarvE calculator provides guidance on the number of pots that are appropriate for wounds of different sizes and conditions.

⌘   The Biosurgical Research Unit in Bridgend will provide education and training on maggot therapy at different venues throughout the UK.

References

Chaffrey R (1997) Case study: larval therapy for an infected insect bite. World Wide Wounds. Accessed on: http//:www.smtl.co.uk/World-Wide-Wounds/1997/october/ LarvalTherapy/ LarvalCaseStudy.html

Evans HA (1997) Treatment of last resort. *Nurs Times* **93**(23): 62–5

Freidman E, Shaharabany M, Ravin S *et al* (1998) Partially purified antibacterial agent from maggots displays a wide range of antibacterial activity. Presented at the International Conference on Biotherapy, Jerusalem, Israel

Gacheru I (1998) A case report: the use of maggots in wound treatment. *Nairobi Hosp Proc* **2**(4): 234–8

Jones M, Champion A (1998) Nature's way. *Nurs Times* **94**(34): 75–6

McLellan NW (1932) The maggot treatment of osteomyelitis. *Can Med Assoc J* **27**: 256–60

Mumcuoglu KY, Lipo M, Ioffe-Uspensky I, Miller J, Galun R (1997) Maggot therapy for gangrene and osteomyelitis. *Harefuah* **132**(5): 323–5, 382

Mumcuoglu KY, Miller J, Mumcuoglu M, Friger M, Tarshis M (2001) Destruction of bacteria in the digestive tract of the maggot of *Lucilia sericata*. *J Med Entomol* **38**(2): 161–6

Namias N, Varela JE, Varas RP, Quintana O, Ward CG (2000) Biodebridement: a case report of maggot therapy for limb salvage after fourth-degree burns. *J Burn Care Rehabil* **21**(3): 254–7

Prete P (1997) Growth effects of *Phaenicia sericata* larval extracts on fibroblasts: mechanism for wound healing by maggot therapy. *Life Sci* **60**(8): 505–10

Rayman A, Stansfield G, Woolard T, Mackie A, Rayman G (1998) Use of larvae in the treatment of the diabetic necrotic foot. *Diab Foot* **1**(1): 7–13

Robinson W (1934) Suggestions to facilitate the use of surgical maggots in suppurative infections. *Am J Surg* **25**: 525

Sherman RA (1998) Maggot debridement in modern medicine. *Infect Med* **15**: 651–6

Sherman RA, Wyle F, Vulpe M, Levsen L, Castillo L (1993) The utility of maggot therapy for treating pressure sores. *J Am Paraplegia Soc* **16**(4): 269–70

Sherman RA, Wyle FA, Thrupp L (1995a) Effects of seven antibiotics on the growth and development of *Phaenicia sericata larvae*. *J Med Entomol* **32**(5): 646–9

Sherman RA, Wyle F, Vulpe M (1995b) Maggot therapy for treating pressure ulcers in spinal cord injury patients. *J Spinal Cord Med* **18**(2): 71–4

Stoddard SR, Sherman RM, Mason BE, Pelsang DJ (1995) Maggot debridement therapy — an alternative treatment for nonhealing ulcers. *J Am Podiatr Med Assoc* **85**(4): 218–21

Thomas S (1998) A wriggling remedy. *Chemistry and Industry* **17**: 680–3

Thomas S, Andrews AM (1999) The effect of hydrogel dressings on maggot development. *J Wound Care* **8**(2): 75–77

Thomas S, Jones M, eds (1999) *The Use of Sterile Maggots in Wound Management*. Wound Care Society, Hungtingdon

Thomas S, Jones M (2001) Wound debridement: evaluating the costs. *Nurs Standard* **15**(22): 59–61

Thomas S, Jones M, Shutler S, Andrews A (1996a) Wound care. All you need to know about... maggots. *Nurs Times* **92**(46): 63–70

Thomas S, Jones M, Shutler S, Jones S (1996b) Using larvae in modern wound management. *J Wound Care* **5**(2): 60–9

Thomas S, Jones M, Andrews AM (1998) The use of larval therapy in wound management. *J Wound Care* **7**(10): 521–4

Thomas S, Andrews AM, Hay NP, Bourgoise S (1999) The anti-microbial activity of maggot secretions: results of a preliminary study. *J Tissue Viabil* **9**(4): 127–32

Turner W (2001) Maggot therapy and diabetic ulcers: a randomized controlled trial. Presentation to the Biosurgical Conference, Bridgend

Wayman J, Nirojogi V, Walker A *et al* (2000) The cost-effectiveness of larval therapy in venous ulcers. *J Tissue Viabil* **10**(3): 91–4

Wayman J, Nirojogi V, Walker A *et al* (2001) The cost-effectiveness of larval therapy in venous ulcers. (Erratum.) *J Tissue Viabil* **11**(1): 5

Part II: The effect of containment on the properties of sterile maggots

A laboratory-based study undertaken to examine the effect of confinement in net bags upon the feeding mechanisms and growth rate of maggots of Lucilia sericata showed that free-range maggots survived better and grew significantly faster than maggots in bags (P<0.005). In a separate study it was also demonstrated that maggots in bags could survive on wound fluid that passed through the net without their having access to any form of solid food. This finding was consistent with clinical experience that suggests that although there may be some aesthetic advantages to the use of maggots in bags, their ability to combat infection or remove necrotic tissue from wounds is greatly reduced.

Many clinical publications have described the therapeutic advantages associated with this unconventional form of treatment, and numerous reviews describing the history, mode of action and clinical evidence for maggot therapy have been produced over the last five years (Morgan, 1995; Thomas *et al*, 1996; Sherman *et al*, 2000). All these publications describe the use of 'free-range' maggots, which are introduced directly into a wound and are allowed to roam freely over the surface.

When applied in this way, the maggots are also able to explore the depths of cavities and sinuses in search of the necrotic material that represents their principal source of nutrient.

Patient acceptance of the technique has generally been very high (Sherman, 1998). However, perhaps not surprisingly, a small proportion of patients and some clinicians find this form of treatment unacceptable because of the so-called 'yuk factor', an understandable reaction to 'creepy-crawlies', particularly those more commonly associated with dirt and disease.

In an attempt to make maggot therapy more acceptable to these individuals, a surgeon in Germany, an enthusiastic advocate of maggot therapy, has described a technique by which maggots are supplied in a sealed bag made from nylon net or polyvinyl alcohol foam (Fleischman, 2001). These bags are applied directly to the wound and held in place with an appropriate secondary dressing.

Depending upon the nature of the material from which the bag is constructed, application and removal is facilitated and the enclosed maggots are either partially or totally obscured from view. If maggots applied in this way could be shown to be as effective as the 'free-range' variety, the use of the bags would appear to offer a significant advantage over the more conventional technique.

The aim of this section is to review the scientific and clinical evidence for the use of maggots in bags and identify the indications for which these may be best suited.

Maggots: mode of action

It has previously been suggested that maggots feed mainly by a process of extra-corporeal digestion (Thomas *et al*, 1996), secreting or excreting proteolytic enzymes into the wound which break down the necrotic tissue into a semiliquid form that the creatures subsequently ingest.

This probably represents an over-simplification of the feeding process, for careful observation of feeding maggots also reveals that the creatures use their mouth hooks (*Figure 3.2*) to rip or tear at their food.

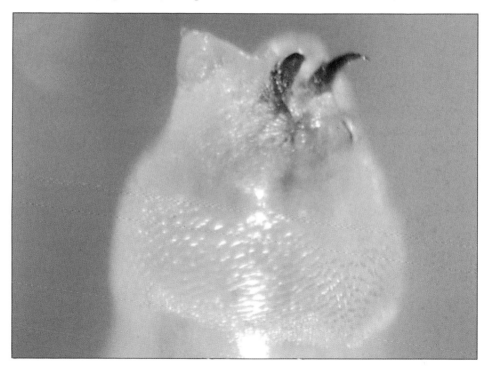

Figure 3.2: Close up of maggot showing mouth hooks in extended position

This activity was graphically described by Stewart (1934) as follows:

> *The process of feeding is characterized by vigorous movements of the head and is not merely a passive act of sucking up fluids… the anterior end of the body is reared up from the tissues and is then brought forcibly down on the surface thereby enabling the strong mouth hooks to tear and cut the tissues.*

The feeding behaviour of maggots of a different but related species of fly was recently captured on camera. Images from the video illustrate the various stages of this process (*Figure 3.3*), although these fail to convey the apparent ferocity with which a maggot appears to attack its food. It must be remembered, however, that this activity takes place on a microscale and is undetectable by the patient.

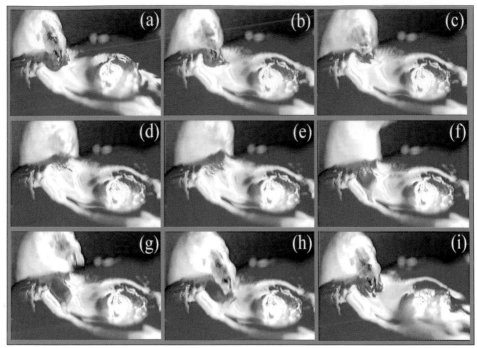

Figure 3.3: Images of maggot feeding: a) and (b) the maggot extends its anterior section and stabs its mouth hooks into the tissue: (c) and (d) it then contracts its body, pulling the mouth hooks backward: (e) and (f) as the hooks tear out of the tissue, the anterior portion of the maggot's body snaps backwards (g) the maggot then stretches forward once again (h) re-extends its mouth hooks, and stabs these downwards once more (i) the entire process then begins again

It is assumed that the scraping or tearing action, first described by Stewart (1934), facilitates penetration of the maggots' proteolytic enzymes, but it has also been shown that the maggots ingest small pieces of tissue released by this process. Microscopic examination of their crops has revealed solid particles of irregular shape up to 75 microns in diameter — presumably produced by the physical destruction of the dead tissue (Stewart, 1934).

Actively feeding maggots also ingest the bacteria associated with this tissue debris and these are killed as they pass through the insects' gut (Robinson and Norwood, 1933, 1934; Mumcuoglu *et al*, 2001). The ingestion and destruction of bacteria in this way probably represents an important part of the observed ability of maggots to combat clinical wound infections (Thomas and Jones, 2000).

The active feeding mechanisms described above obviously cannot take place if maggots are confined within net or foam bags, although it is possible that their secretions may pass out through the wall of the bag and solubilize the necrotic material with which it comes into contact.

Some of this liquefied material may find its way back into the bag to be digested by the maggots, but a significant proportion probably does not. As the quantity of enzymes produced by a maggot increases as the creature grows, it follows that the rate of wound cleansing will accelerate with time as the maggots increase in size. If the growth of confined maggots is inhibited, the wound cleansing process, if it takes place at all, is likely to be retarded and much less effective than with free-range maggots.

Larval feeding studies

In order to compare the effect of containment upon the growth rate and development of free-range and confined maggots, some simple feeding studies were conducted.

Comparative growth rates of free and contained maggots

Six net bags were prepared, each measuring approximately 7.5cm x 7.5cm and containing twenty sterile second instar maggots from a common source. These bags were placed onto 10g portions of pigs' liver in Petri dishes and left in a warm dark place for forty-eight hours.

A similar number of dishes were set up containing twenty maggots from the same batch that were allowed to move freely over the liver. After forty-eight hours the maggots in each dish were counted and weighed and then the entire experiment was repeated a second time with five net bags containing a second batch of maggots (*Table 3.1*).

Table 3.1: Effect of confinement upon maggot growth

No of survivors		Total weight of maggots (g)		Average weight of maggots (g)	
In bags	Free range	In bags	Free range	In bags	Free range
0*	17		0.52		0.031
0*	18		0.37		0.021
11	17	0.16	0.2	0.015	0.012
13	16	0.19	0.37	0.015	0.023
12	15	0.15	0.24	0.013	0.016
19	16	0.17	0.18	0.009	0.011
17	19	0.19	0.34	0.011	0.018
18	13	0.24	0.35	0.013	0.027
15	20	0.22	0.47	0.015	0.024
13	16	0.16	0.32	0.012	0.020
13	18	0.17	0.41	0.013	0.023
Total 131	Total 185	Total 1.65	Total 3.77	Average 0.013	Average 0.020

*excluded from calculations

In two of the bags the maggots failed to survive. Although the reason for this is not clear, it is possible that they failed to gain access to sufficient food in the early stages of their development. The results of these two studies, excluding the two bags in which all the maggots died, indicate that the difference between the survival rates of maggots in bags (73%) compared with free-range maggots (84%) just failed to achieve significance at the 95% level (P=0.06). Highly significant differences were recorded between these groups for both the total weight of maggots (1.65g for the maggots in bags and 3.77g for the free-range maggots; P=0.0004) and their average weight (0.013g and 0.02g; P=0.0016).

This difference is important because in a clinical situation the increase in the weight of a maggot is determined by the amount of necrotic material it ingests. The bigger it gets the more enzymes it is able to produce and the more necrotic tissue it is able to remove. This simple study suggests that maggots with unrestricted access to a food source will ingest twice as much dead tissue as those confined within a net bag in a comparable period of time. In simple terms, they will cleanse a wound at least twice as fast.

In fact, these results may actually overestimate the wound cleansing effect of confined maggots. Although the results of this simple study appear to suggest that maggots may be absorbing externally digested food through the bag wall as suggested previously, it is possible that they are simply feeding upon blood or other fluid lost from the liver as it passes through the nylon mesh.

In order to examine the ability of the larvae to survive upon tissue fluid in this way, a second study was undertaken in which maggots in bags were fed on a liquid diet using a wound model consisting of a stainless steel plate 200mm x 200mm, mounted horizontally, bearing a central circular recess 2mm deep and 50mm diameter. In the base of this recess is a narrow channel 1.25mm deep (*Figure 3.4*). In normal use, test fluid is applied to this channel via a port in the undersurface of the plate by means of a syringe pump, and taken up by a dressing applied to the upper surface. Full details of the construction and use of this equipment have been published previously (Thomas and Fram, 2001).

For the purposes of this study, foetal bovine serum was used as a wound exudate substitute and this was applied to the plate using the syringe pump with a flow rate of 0.5ml per hour. A piece of filter paper was placed over the channel to act as a spreader layer, and a bag containing twenty maggots with an average weight of 0.001g was placed on top and covered with five non-woven swabs to draw fluid up through the nylon mesh and absorb any excess. A second wound model was set up in an identical manner.

After forty-eight hours the bags were removed (*Figure 3.5*) and the number of maggots in both were counted, weighed and compared with values obtained with forty similar free-range maggots that were allowed to feed on liver in the normal way.

Within the two bags a total of twenty-seven maggots survived with a mean weight of 0.007g. This compared with a mean weight of 0.023g for the thirty surviving free-range maggots.

The results confirmed that the maggots in the bags were able to obtain sufficient nutrient from a protein-rich liquid diet to increase their body weight by a factor of seven in forty-eight hours, but this was substantially less than the increase recorded for free-range maggots which increased to twenty-three times their original weight in the same time period. Nevertheless, the results confirm that in the clinical situation, maggots in bags placed on to moist wounds could survive and grow on exudate alone without necessarily producing any wound-debriding effect.

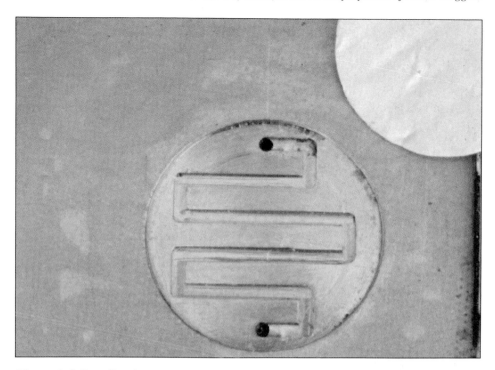

Figure 3.4: Details of wound model

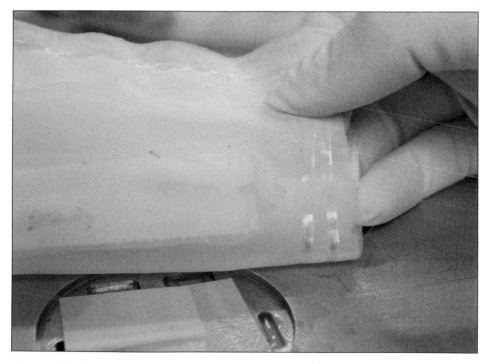

Figure 3.5: Removal of bag after forty-eight hours

The clinical relevance of this observation may be illustrated by reference to the following case history.

Case history

An eighty-year-old man with complex medical problems, including a colostomy, was admitted to hospital with a fractured femur and a long-standing, heavily-discharging, infected abscess in his right groin which was methicillin-resistant *Staphylococcus aureus* (MRSA) positive. The wound was approximately 30mm x 10mm and full of necrotic tissue.

As a result of the difficult location of the wound, it was decided to apply maggots in a fine mesh bag and hold them in place with a hydrocolloid sheet in the centre of which a large hole had been cut to form a border. An absorbent pad, held in place with surgical tape, completed the dressing, which was left in place for three days.

Upon removal, it was noted that although the maggots had increased a little in size (*Figure 3.6*), there was no detectable change in the condition of the wound, which was still full of thick yellow slough (*Figure 3.7*).

At this stage, despite the difficult location it was decided to switch to free-range maggots, which were applied using the standard technique (Thomas *et al*, 1996). Two days later, when the dressing was removed, a marked difference was detected in the wound, which was filled with actively feeding maggots (*Figure 3.8*). These had digested a significant amount of the slough and begun to reveal the full extent of the cavity (*Figure 3.9*). Further applications of maggots were made until the wound was slough-free, at which time it was dressed with alginate packing. Swabs of the wound taken after maggot therapy revealed that the MRSA had also been eliminated.

These clinical results are consistent with our previous experience involving maggots in bags (unpublished results). They support the hypothesis derived from the laboratory study that the creatures can grow by feeding upon exudate produced by a wound, without making any significant impact on the amount of slough present.

Conclusion

Historically, the Biosurgical Research Unit has received a number of requests for maggots in bags (LarvE Bags). These have been supplied on the understanding that the effectiveness of this application system has not been proven and, as such, treatment outcomes must be evaluated critically, for published clinical experiences with free-range maggots cannot be applied to those contained in a bag.

Maggot therapy is very cost-effective when used correctly, but as the unit cost of a container of maggots is not insignificant, the extensive use of maggots in bags represents a significant waste of resources if, as we believe, their effectiveness is reduced significantly in this presentation. There is also a concern that clinicians who have not previously used maggots will purchase the new formulation, find that it does not perform as well as expected, and be put off using maggots in the future.

Occasionally, situations will arise when free-range maggots cannot be used because of the nature or the position of the wound or its proximity to other structures or body orifices. In these situations the use of the bags may be appropriate. Also, this presentation may be acceptable to an individual who simply cannot cope with the idea of maggots crawling freely in his/her wound. It must be emphasized, however, that in both these situations the advantages of convenience and increased patient or doctor acceptability will be offset by a greatly reduced speed of action. It must also be remembered that the use of bags presents practical problems of their own, particularly if they are to be applied like a patchwork quilt to extensive or circumferential leg ulcers.

In summary, although LarvE Bags will continue to be available on request for those who require them for specific situations where the use of free-range maggots may be inappropriate, we would not at this time advocate their more widespread general use either on the basis of cost or clinical efficacy.

Key points

⌘ Despite its widespread use and proven cost-effectiveness, some patients and clinicians still find the idea of maggot therapy unacceptable. It has therefore been suggested that presenting them in some form of 'tea-bag' would overcome these aesthetic problems while facilitating application and removal.

⌘ Laboratory studies indicate that even on relatively flat or open wounds, the feeding mechanisms and the growth rate of maggots applied in this way are impaired, compared with the 'free-range' variety.

⌘ The many clinical papers that describe the use of free-range maggots cannot and should not be assumed to be equally applicable to maggots applied in net or foam bags.

The authors would like to thank Thierry Berrod and Mona Lisa Productions, Lyon, France, for permission to use the video images and Mr Peter Phillips, Deputy Director of SMTL for statistical advice.

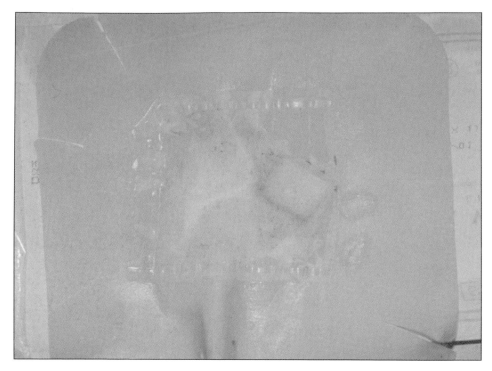

Figure 3.6: Bag removed from wound containing partially grown maggots

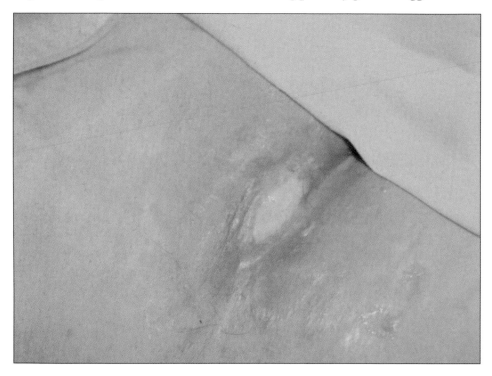

Figure 3.7: Wound after removal of bag, still full of slough

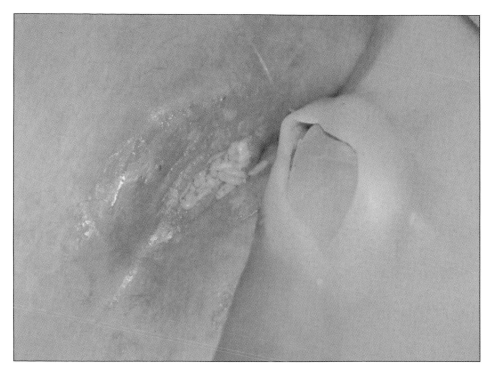

Figure 3.8: Wound after two days of treatment with free-range maggots

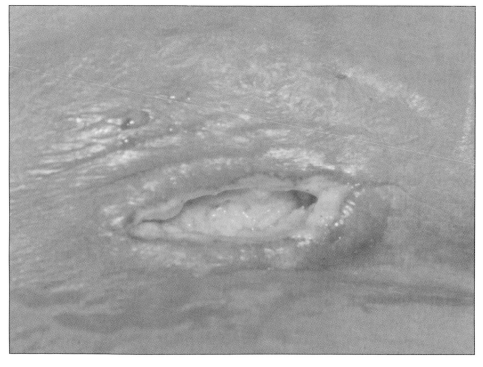

Figure 3.9: Wound after removal of maggots

References

Fleischman W (2001) Presentation to Biosurgical Conference. Biosurgical Research Unit, Bridgend (unpublished)

Morgan D (1995) Myiasis: the rise and fall of maggot therapy. *J Tissue Viabil* **5**(2): 43–51

Mumcuoglu KY, Miller J, Mumcuoglu M, Friger M, Tarshis M (2001) Destruction of bacteria in the digestive tract of the maggot of *Lucilia sericata* (Diptera: Calliphoridae). *J Med Entomol* **38**(2): 161–6

Robinson W, Norwood VH (1933) The role of surgical maggots in the disinfection of osteomyelitis and other infected wounds. *J Bone Joint Surg* **15**: 409–12

Robinson W, Norwood VH (1934) Destruction of pyogenic bacteria in the alimentary tract of surgical maggots implanted in infected wounds. *J Lab Clin Med* **19**: 581–6

Sherman RA, Hall MJ, Thomas S (2000) Medicinal maggots: an ancient remedy for some contemporary afflictions. *Annu Rev Entomol* **45**: 55–81

Sherman RA (1998) Maggot debridement in modern medicine. *Infections in Medicine* **15**: 651–6

Stewart MA (1934) The role of *Lucilia sericata* Meig. larvae in osteomyelitis wounds. *Ann Trop Med Parasitol* **28**: 445–60

Thomas S, Jones M (2000) *Maggots and the Battle Against MRSA*. Surgical Materials Testing Laboratory, Bridgend

Thomas S, Fram P (2001) The development of a novel technique for predicting the exudate handling properties of modern wound dressing. *J Tissue Viabil* **11**(4): 145–60

Thomas S, Jones M, Shutler S, Jones S (1996) Using larvae in modern wound management. *J Wound Care* **5**(2): 60–9

4

Improving diagnosis of malignant leg ulcers in the community

Rachael Walsh

Over 80% of all leg ulcer patients are cared for in the community by district and practice nurses, or by a relative who may or may not be adequately instructed or supervised. Many patients have never been referred for a specialist opinion, although their ulcers have been in existence for many years. This chapter discusses the current lack of community leg ulcer nurse specialists who could perform biopsies on non-healing wounds and thus reduce the amount of unnecessary hospital referrals. In turn, this would speed referral times to hospital of patients with malignant leg ulcers.

Before discussing the aetiology of leg ulceration it is worth defining the term 'leg ulcer'. The following definition, which has been used in an epidemiological study (Dale *et al*, 1983), is useful because it is simple and makes no assumption as to the cause of the ulceration:

> *A leg ulcer is a loss of skin below the knee on the leg or foot which takes more than six weeks to heal.*
>
> Dale *et al*, 1983

This definition is clear, concise and non-judgmental and will be the definition used in this chapter when discussing leg ulcers.

Chronic leg ulcers

Chronic leg ulcers are an important health problem in the UK. Leg ulcers affect 1–2% of the adult population and account for 1% of dermatology referrals (Gawkrodger, 1997). Leg ulcers principally affect elderly people and cost the NHS up to £600m per year (Wilson, 1989). However, Morison and Moffatt (1995) argue that this is almost certainly an overestimate. As part of a European study of the cost of venous disease, the Office of Health Economics estimated the cost in the UK of venous disease to have been £294m in 1989 (Laing, 1992). This is 2% of total healthcare spending in the UK. A high proportion of this is estimated to have been the cost of district nursing services.

In Western countries, ten in every 1000 of the adult population are likely to have a chronic leg ulcer at some time in their lives (Dale *et al*, 1983). Other studies, such as Callam *et al* (1985), Cornwall *et al* (1986) and Nelzen *et al* (1994), found that approximately 60–80% of chronic leg ulcers had a venous component, and 10–30% were associated with arterial insufficiency (this includes patients with diabetes and peripheral vascular disease). The last main group consists of patients with 'mixed' ulcers (approximately 20%), where venous, arterial, rheumatoid arthritis and other diseases play a part. Although malignant leg ulcers are rare, an existing ulcer may become malignant or an existing skin tumour may become ulcerated.

The care of patients with possible malignancy is a neglected area in chronic leg ulcer management. In a detailed literature review, using the main databases, Medline, Cinahl and Bandolier, only two articles specifically related to leg ulcers and malignancy were found (Yang *et al*, 1996; Taylor *et al*, 1997).

Studies have showed that most ulcers are cared for by the general practitioner: 67% in the Lothian and Forth Valley Study (Callam *et al*, 1987) and 78% in a study of Northwick Park (Cornwall *et al*, 1986). In these cases, the principal carer was the district nurse, even when patients were attending hospital out-patient clinics. In the Cornwall *et al* (1986) study, 69% of ulcers were being dressed at home, 48% by the district nurse and 21% by a relative or patient. The clinical management of leg ulcers, therefore, falls to a primary care discipline, with most being cared for in the community.

Cullum and Last (1993), in their survey of leg ulcer management in the Wirral, found that 19% of initial diagnoses of a leg ulcer were undertaken by nurses. Cullum (1994) was concerned that not all patients with leg ulcers were given the benefit of a medical examination and a medical diagnosis. If this is the case, there is a need to train community nurses adequately to undertake comprehensive nursing assessments and know when to refer to GPs or consultants.

Callam *et al* (1987) obtained information on the clinical history of a sample of 600 of the 1477 leg ulcer cases identified in the original study (Callam *et al*, 1987). Forty-five per cent of patients reported episodes of ulceration for more than ten years. Half of current ulcers had been open for more than nine months, 20% had not healed after two years and 8% were still open after five years. Similar figures were reported by Cornwall *et al* (1986), with 50% of ulcers being present for over a year.

These two studies highlighted slow healing rates. Moffatt *et al* (1992), however, reported healing rates of 67% of venous leg ulcers within twelve weeks. These results are supported by Stevens *et al* (1997) who reported similar healing rates (66%) and can be further substantiated by Simon *et al*'s (1996) study which reported that the best healing rates at three months was 65% in patients treated in community clinics. Nelson (1998) suggests that healing rates for leg ulcers should be measured at intervals over a period of probably more than twelve weeks. This suggestion is suitable only if there is evidence of wound healing and not stasis or deterioration occurring at these intervals.

It is worth mentioning that without a randomized control trial, healing rates are difficult to interpret because of the many confounding variables. These include ulcer type, size and duration.

The extent of the delayed ulcer healing rates may have been because of a reduction in the healing capacity of the skin itself, as reduced activity of macrophages within elderly people has been identified and extensively reviewed (Dalziel and Bickers, 1992; Mast, 1992).

Many studies confirm that the number of patients with leg ulcerations who are referred for a specialist opinion is low. Cornwall *et al* (1986) reported that 62% of patients had never seen a specialist. Later, Cullum and Last (1993) found that only 41% of patients had ever been referred to hospital.

It is difficult to judge the appropriateness of these figures as there is no 'gold standard' referral rate and referral may have been inappropriate or refused by the patient in a large number of cases. However, seventy-seven patients in Cullum and Last's (1993) study who had leg ulcers for six months or more had never been referred. The importance of referring patients with non-healing or idiosyncratic ulceration needs to be emphasized to GPs and nurses as specialist assessment of a patient may isolate unrecognized factors such as arterial insufficiency or carcinoma (Ackroyd and Young, 1983).

In a study carried out in 1991 (Roe *et al*, 1993), 63% of nurses would refer a patient for a medical opinion if the person's ulcer was not healing. However, GPs tend to view the nurse as the leg ulcer specialist and devolve treatment options to them; therefore, referral to the GP may be insufficient and further referral to a consultant may be necessary.

It is evident that all patients with chronic leg ulcers require an accurate medical diagnosis and comprehensive nursing assessment in order that the most appropriate care can be planned and delivered. Whatever the underlying pathology appears to be, it is important to rule out the more unusual causes of ulceration, such as malignancy.

Tests required to exclude the more uncommon causes of ulceration are beyond the role of the nurse, but as most patients in the UK are assessed and treated by community nurses, the nurse has a vital role to play in referring patients for further detailed assessment. It is perhaps worth considering the role of community-led leg ulcer clinics in undertaking a biopsy of suspicious or non-healing ulcers and, therefore, speeding up the appropriate referral rate. However, there appears to be no information on this particular area of leg ulcer management.

Before the Royal College of Nursing (RCN) guidelines, *The Management of Patients with Venous Leg Ulcers* (RCN, 1998) and the Scottish Intercollegiate Guidelines Network (SIGN) guidelines, *The Care of Patients with Chronic Leg Ulcers* (SIGN, 1998), there were no published clinical guidelines on the management of leg ulcers based on a systematic literature review. However, there were consensus-based guidelines from the British Association of Dermatologists (Douglas and Simpson, 1995). The Scottish Health Purchasing Information Centre had also completed an evidence-based report on leg ulcer care (Scottish Health Purchasing Information Centre, 1996).

Clinical guidelines

Clinical guidelines are usually defined as 'systematically developed statements to assist practitioner and patient decisions about appropriate health care for specific circumstances' (Institute for Medicine, 1992). They are made up of recommendations for the care of clients with a particular condition, in this case, leg ulcers.

The guidelines developed by SIGN (1998) have been adapted for local use in the author's primary care trust as it makes economic sense for trusts to use guidelines that have been developed at a national level, are based on systematic reviews of research literature and appear more detailed in their content and more prescriptive in their recommendations than the RCN (1998) guidelines. However, at present there is insufficient high-quality research to provide grade A recommendations (grade A requires at least one randomized control trial as part of a body of literature which is generally consistent in most acceptable studies).

Guidelines are viewed as an important tool in the quest to promote evidence-based practice. They are useful because they synthesize evidence into clear recommendations for practice, thereby helping to overcome some of the practical difficulties faced by practitioners in the reality of the clinical context.

According to the SIGN (1998) guidelines, if the ulcer is non-healing after twelve weeks or appears abnormal, the patient should be referred for a biopsy. This recommendation is based on evidence obtained from expert committee reports or opinions and not on any quality studies or trials. However, as already highlighted by Cornwall *et al* (1986), Cullum and Last (1993) and Roe *et al* (1993), many patients are not being referred to specialists, such as dermatologists or vascular surgeons. If they are referred, many are not referred until after the twelve weeks of active treatment.

It is the author's view that if ulcers are not responding to treatment after eight weeks, we should be referring patients sooner to specialists as appointments to see specialists can take longer than a week. In addition, patients referred to vascular consultants may not be seen until at least one to two months later, exceeding the recommended twelve-week reassessment. Perhaps nurses in community leg ulcer clinics with specialist training should be undertaking biopsies to eliminate uncommon and rare causes of ulceration before hospital referrals.

The appearance of the edge and base of the ulcer can indicate the stage of healing and may suggest complications such as malignancy. The incidence of malignancy indicates the need for the assessment to include a biopsy in unusual or non-healing wounds. Yang *et al* (1996) reported positive biopsy rates as high as 4.4% and Taylor *et al* (1997) identified twelve malignancies in less than 200 leg ulcer patients.

As previously mentioned, malignancy is an uncommon cause of ulceration, but this complication should not be overlooked in patients whose ulcers fail to respond to treatment (Ackroyd and Young, 1983).

The community leg ulcer service in Salford is supported by a weekly consultant clinic. All patients referred to the service are initially seen by a specialist nurse or consultant. The increase in the number of malignant leg ulcers referred to the service has raised the awareness of the need for tissue biopsy for all venous ulcers that fail to respond to treatment.

In a survey, within a year, twelve patients with diagnosed malignant ulceration presented to a community leg ulcer clinic (Taylor *et al*, 1997; Taylor, 1998). Of these, seven basal cell carcinomas and five squamous cell carcinomas (two cases of Marjolin's ulcers) were diagnosed.

Leg ulcer malignancies

Tumours may arise as thickenings in actinic keratosis (sun wart), discrete, rough, premalignant surfaced lesions. They are pink or grey and seldom exceed 1cm in diameter. Transition to squamous cell carcinoma occurs if a lesion enlarges, ulcerates or bleeds. However, the tumour may start as an ulcer with a granulating base and an indurated edge. It is worth discussing the various types of skin tumours which may arise on the leg and may be seen, misdiagnosed or inappropriately referred.

Squamous cell carcinoma

This is a common tumour (*Figure 4.1*). It often arises in skin damaged by long-term ultraviolet radiation, X-rays and infrared rays. Other carcinogens include tar, pitch, mineral oils and inorganic arsenic. A squamous cell carcinoma can develop in a chronic venous ulcer and is known as Marjolin's ulcer. The condition is rare but should be suspected if the ulcer has an unusual appearance, including overgrowth of tissue at the base or at the ulcer's margins. Squamous cell carcinomas occur in people over fifty-five years of age and are more common in males. More aggressive ulcerating forms are seen developing at the edge of ulcers, in scars and at sites of radiation damage. Metastases are found in 10% or more of these cancers (Gawkrodger, 1997). Marjolin's ulcer is confirmed by a biopsy and histological examination.

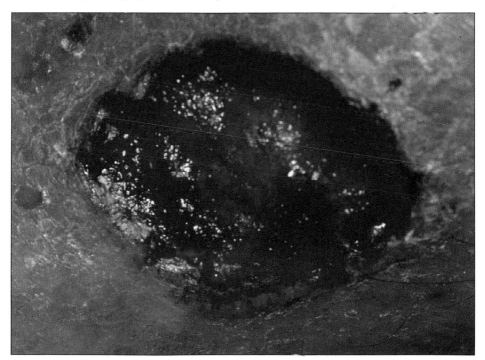

Figure 4.1: Squamous cell carcinoma

Malignant melanoma

Malignant melanoma attracts a large amount of attention because it is often lethal (*Figure 4.2*). The incidence in the white population in the UK and USA is doubling approximately every ten years. In Scotland, the incidence is now ten in 100,000 people each year. It accounts for 50% of all UK malignant skin tumour cases, shows a female preponderance and is commonest on the lower leg (Gawkrodger, 1997). Malignant melanoma is unlikely to be mistaken for a venous ulcer, but it can bear a superficial resemblance to Kaposi's sarcoma.

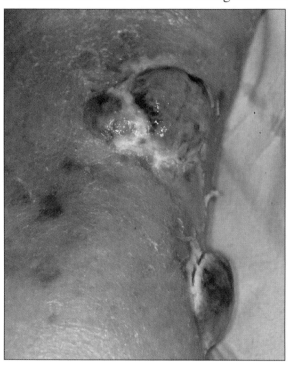

Figure 4.2: Malignant melanoma — advanced — note the melanin deposits in the skin

Eighty per cent of invasive melanomas are preceded by a superficial and radial growth phase, shown clinically as an expanding, irregularly pigmented macule or plaques. Most are multicoloured, their margins irregular with notches. They are usually confined to the epidermis and uppermost dermis, but eventually invade deeper and metastasize. The life expectancy of a patient diagnosed with malignant melanoma can vary depending on the age of the patient, the site and depth and the clinical stage of the tumour. For example, if the tumour is stage one, the five-year survival rate is 75%, but at stage three this figure is only 0–5% (Mackie, 1995).

Kaposi's sarcoma

Kaposi's sarcoma may be multifocal. There are two types: classic, and that associated with immunosuppression. Classic sarcoma is mostly seen in Africans and elderly Jews of European origin (Hunter *et al*, 1996). The tumours are usually on the feet and ankles. Initially, they are dark blue/purple macules, progressing to tumours and plaques which ulcerate. Tumours may metastasize to lymph nodes and spread to internal organs. Oedema of the legs may be severe. If a lesion presents on the ankle, it could be misdiagnosed by community nurses as being related to venous insufficiency. The life expectancy is five to nine years.

Kaposi's sarcoma and immunosuppression have recently become well known because of the association with acquired immunodeficiency syndrome

(AIDS). Lesions may occur anywhere and are initially bruise-like. However, lesions tend to occur on the trunk, head or neck areas and arise frequently in the mouth. The prognosis of AIDS patients with Kaposi's sarcoma is poor. The life expectancy is about one year (Hunter *et al*, 1996).

Intraepidermal carcinoma (Bowen's disease)

Intraepidermal carcinoma (Bowen's disease) usually consists of single, slowly expanding pink scaly plaques which take years to reach a diameter of a few centimetres (*Figure 4.3*). Their border is sharply defined, with reniform projections and notches. These lesions occasionally change into an invasive squamous cell carcinoma. Intraepidermal carcinoma is often mistaken for psoriasis, discoid eczema or a superficial basal cell carcinoma. For community nurses who are unfamiliar with dermatological disorders, the intraepidermal carcinoma can be vesicular and weeping and can look like an area of ulceration or over-granulation.

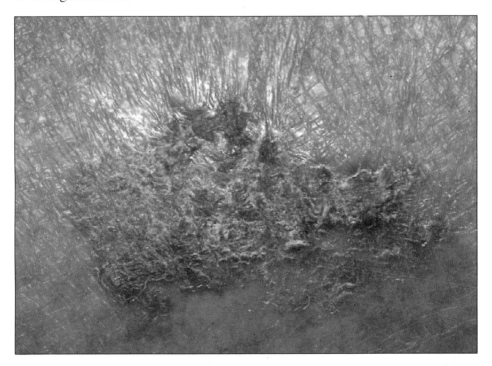

Figure 4.3: Bowen's disease on the calf — a five-year history

Basal cell carcinoma

Basal cell carcinoma is the most common form of skin cancer (Hunter *et al*, 1996) (*Figure 4.4*). Lesions invade locally but, for practical purposes, never metastasize. Prolonged sun exposure is the most common factor. Basal cell carcinoma is mostly found in Caucasians living near the equator. They may also occur in scars caused by X-rays, vaccinations or trauma (Hunter *et al*, 1996).

An early lesion is a small, glistening, translucent, skin-coloured papule which slowly enlarges leaving an ulcer with a rolled pearly edge. Cicatricial lesions are another type causing ulceration and crusting followed by fibrosis and may mimic scar tissue. The five-year cure rate for all types of basal cell carcinoma is over 95%, but regular follow-up is necessary to detect local recurrence (Hunter *et al*, 1996).

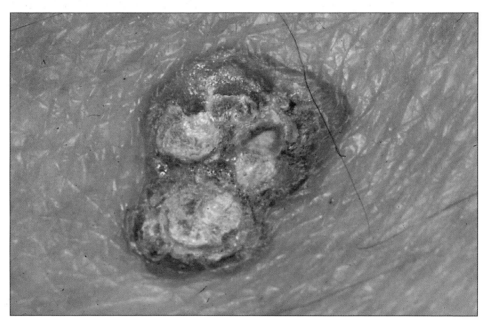

Figure 4.4: Basal cell carcinoma — note the round, rolled edge

Little is known or published in relation to management of malignant leg ulcers. As survival rates for each of the malignancies discussed are mostly poor, it becomes increasingly apparent that there is a need for quicker diagnosis, confirmed by biopsy and referral for appropriate treatment.

Biopsy

As previously mentioned, neoplastic ulcers or neoplastic change in pre-existing ulcers are uncommon, but may give rise to diagnostic difficulty. As suggested in the SIGN (1998) guidelines, a referral for biopsy should be considered if the appearance of the ulcer is atypical or there is deterioration or failure to progress after twelve weeks of active treatment.

The cost of a small biopsy can vary depending on the examinations required, ie. between £20 and £30 (the cost can increase to £600 for electromicroscopy) (Chief Technician at the Manchester Royal Infirmary, personal communication). Most common malignancies, depending on their clinical stage, such as malignant melanoma, basal cell carcinoma and small cell carcinoma, can be detected on routine histopathology examinations.

However, the use of a bacteriological swab to sample the flora of a wound is taken for granted. The cost of a swab for culture and sensitivity is approximately £15, with a further £5 per further examination. When comparing the costs of a biopsy with the detection of malignancy and the cost of a wound swab taken for diagnosis of wound infection, it appears to be equivalent.

In the absence of clinical signs of infection, eg. cellulitis, there is no indication for routine bacteriological swabbing and yet it is common practice for clinicians to swab chronic leg ulcers 'to find out what might be there'. Routine swabbing is not justified by the literature, and may be an expensive waste of resources. All ulcers will be colonized by microorganisms at some point, and colonization in itself is not associated with delayed healing (Trengove *et al*, 1996). The most important limitation of the swab is that it only samples the surface of the wound. The methods of swabbing are diverse and often lack a rational basis (Gilchrist, 1996).

Biopsy, followed by suitable processing (Heggars *et al*, 1969; Lawrence and Ameen, 1998) can overcome this difficulty. However, the method requires skilled expertise to ensure minimal pain is inflicted on the patient as it is an invasive procedure. Some authors, notably Robson (1991), have suggested that biopsy is the 'gold standard' and the only method that will give reliable results when defining infection. Heggars *et al* (1969) and Stotts (1995) support this view. The biggest single drawback would seem to be that biopsy is not routinely performed in the community where most chronic leg ulcer care takes place. Most community nurses are unfamiliar with the technique or are not authorized to carry it out and, therefore, it is confined to hospitals or specialist centres.

Recommendations for practice

There is a need to address the training needs of community nurses regarding leg ulcer management. As highlighted by Cullum (1994), the initial diagnosis and management of leg ulcers were attributed to nurses with little or no specialist training. Considering 1–2% of the population will have a leg ulcer at least once in their lifetime, it is worrying that formal training of community nurses has, until recently, been overlooked. Courses, such as the ENB N18 Care of Patients with Leg Ulcers, offer evidence-based literature and structured training.

As an alternative to training district nurses to a high level of expertise in leg ulcer management, a smaller number of trained specialist nurses could be provided who might carry out a full leg ulcer assessment, including a biopsy in the community setting. Service provision and training issues would have to be addressed at a local level. Changes in the health service should encourage the development of innovative approaches and professional development. There is an increasing demand for services to bridge the gap between the acute and community services and the development of community-based initiatives to propose leg ulcer specialist nurses to perform biopsies. This could potentially reduce the number of referrals to hospital-based leg ulcer clinics while speeding up the appropriate referrals once the diagnosis has been confirmed.

Rachael Walsh

Conclusion

As highlighted by the lack of literature available, the diagnosis of patients with suspicious or non-healing ulcers is a neglected area of leg ulcer management which needs to be addressed. Over 80% of all leg ulcer patients are cared for in the community by district and practice nurses, or by a relative who may or may not be adequately instructed or supervised (Cornwall *et al*, 1986). Many patients have never been referred for a specialist opinion, although their ulcers have been open for many years. Those who are referred to hospital outpatient clinics may be seen by a variety of specialists, including dermatologists and vascular surgeons. However, despite there being many places of clinical excellence, overall provision of specialist care is patchy in the UK (Gilliland and Wolfe, 1991).

The paucity of good research in the field of leg ulcer management and the need for clinical effectiveness, means it is more pertinent for community nurses to have sound evidence-based knowledge. Unfortunately, there is no evidence available on this area of leg ulcer management. Hopefully, in the future, it may be explored in clinical studies and deemed clinically cost-effective for both practitioners and service providers.

Key points

⌘ Leg ulcers have been estimated to cost 2% of health expenditure in the UK.

⌘ The clinical care of many cases of leg ulcers is done in the community.

⌘ Many studies confirm a low referral rate to specialist skin ulcer units.

⌘ Leg ulcers that do not respond to treatment in eight weeks should be referred to either a dermatologist or vascular surgeon.

⌘ Malignancy, an uncommon cause of ulceration, should be considered when an ulcer does not respond to treatment.

⌘ It is hoped that more research and greater nurse expertise may reduce the number of patients referred to specialist ulcer clinics.

References

Ackroyd JS, Young AE (1983) Leg ulcers that do not heal. *Br Med J* **286**: 207–8

Callam MJ, Ruckley CV, Harper DR, Dale JJ (1985) Chronic ulceration of the leg: extent of the problem and provision of care. *Br Med J* **240**: 1855–6

Callam MJ, Dale JJ, Harper DR, Ruckley CV (1987) Arterial disease in chronic leg ulceration: an underestimated hazard? Lothian and Forth Valley leg ulcer study. *Br Med J* **294**: 929–31

Cornwall J, Dore CJ, Lewis JD (1986) Leg ulcers: epidemiology and aetiology. *Br J Surg* **73**: 693–6

Cullum N, Last S (1993) The prevalence, characteristics and management of leg ulcers in a UK community. Second European Conference on Advances in Wound Management, Harrogate

Cullum N (1994) *The Nursing Management of Leg Ulcers in the Community: A Critical Review of Research*. Department of Nursing, University of Liverpool

Dale J, Callam M, Ruckley C, Harper D, Berrey PN (1983) Chronic ulcers of the leg: a study of prevalence in a Scottish community. *Health Bull* **41**: 310–4

Dalziel KL, Bickers DR (1992) Skin ageing. In: Brocklehurst JC, Tallis RC, Fillit HM, eds. *Textbook of Geriatric Medicine and Gerontology*. 4th edn. Churchill Livingstone, Edinburgh: 898–921

Douglas DW, Simpson NB (1995) Guidelines for the management of chronic venous leg ulceration. Report of a multidisciplinary workshop. *Br J Dermatol* **132**: 446–52

Gawkrodger D (1997) *Dermatology: An Illustrated Colour Text*. 2nd edn. Churchill Livingstone, London

Gilchrist B (1996) Sampling bacterial flora: a review of the literature. *J Wound Care* **5**(8): 384–8

Gilliland EL, Wolfe JHN (1991) Leg ulcers. *Br Med J* **303**: 776–9

Heggars JP, Robson MC, Ristroph JD (1969) A rapid method of performing quantitative wound cultures. *Mil Med* **134**(9): 666–7

Hunter J, Savin J, Dahl M (1996) *Clinical Dermatology*. 2nd edn. Blackwell Science, Oxford

Institute for Medicine (1992) *Guidelines for Clinical Practice: From Development to Use*. National Academic Press, Washington

Laing W (1992) *Chronic Venous Diseases of the Leg*. Office of Health Economics, London

Lawrence JC, Ameen H (1998) Swabs and other sampling techniques. J *Wound Care* **7**(5): 232–3

Mackie RM (1995) Melanoma. *Br Med Bull* **5**(3): 523–760

Mast BA (1992) The skin. In: Cohen IK, Diegelmann RF, Lynd Bland WJ, eds. *Wound Healing: Biochemical and Clinical Aspects*. WB Saunders, Philadelphia: 344–55

Moffatt CJ, Franks PJ, Oldroyd M *et al* (1992) Community clinics for leg ulcers and their impact on healing. *Br Med J* **305**: 1389–92

Morison M, Moffatt C (1995) *A Colour Guide to the Assessment and Management of Leg Ulcers*. 2nd edn. Mosby, London

Nelson EA (1998) The evidence in support of compression bandaging. *J Wound Care* **7**(3): 148–50

Nelzen O, Bergqvist D, Lindbagen A (1994) Venous and non-venous leg ulcers: clinical history and appearance in a population study. *Br J Surg* **81**: 182–7

Robson M (1991) Plastic surgery. In: Heggars J, Robson M, eds. *Quantitative Bacteriology: Its Role in the Armamentarium of the Surgeon*. CRC Press, Boca Raton, Florida

Roe B, Luker KA, Cullum NA, Griffiths JM, Kenrick M (1993) Assessment, prevention and monitoring of chronic leg ulcers in the community: report of a survey. *J Clin Nurs* **2**(5): 299–306

Royal College of Nursing (1998) *The Management of Patients with Venous Leg Ulcers*. RCN Publishing, London

Scottish Health Purchasing Information Centre (1996) *Leg Ulcers*. The Scottish Health Purchasing Centre, Aberdeen

Scottish Intercollegiate Guidelines Network (1998) *The Care of Patients with Chronic Leg Ulcers*. SIGN, Edinburgh

Simon D, Freak L, Kinsella A *et al* (1996) Community leg ulcer clinics: a comparative study in two health authorities. *Br Med J* **312**: 1648–51

Stevens J, Franks P, Harrington MA (1997) Community/hospital leg ulcer service. *J Wound Care* **6**(9): 62–8

Stotts N (1995) Determination of bacterial burden in wounds. *Adv Wound Care* **8**(8): 46–52

Taylor A, Marcuson R, Whiteby C (1997) The importance of tissue biopsy for non-healing leg ulcers (abstract). In: Leaper D *et al*, eds. *New Approaches to the Management of Chronic Wounds*. Proceedings of the 7th European Conference on Advances in Wound Management, Macmillan, London

Taylor A (1998) The importance of tissue biopsy in non-healing leg ulcers. *J Tissue Viabil* **8**(3): 32

Trengove N, Stacey M, McGechie D (1996) Qualitative bacteriology and leg ulcer healing. *J Wound Care* **5**(6): 277–80

Wilson E (1989) Just briefly: prevention and treatment of leg ulcers. *Health Trends* **21**: 97

Yang D, Morrison BD, Vandongen YK, Singh A, Stacey MC (1996) Malignancy in chronic leg ulcers. *Med J Aust* **164**(12): 718–20

5

Pressure ulcer classification: The systems and the pitfalls

Linda Russell

The classification of pressure ulcers constitutes an essential part of patient assessment and forms a baseline on which to monitor patients' progress and measure the outcomes of care. Four classification systems — Torrance, National Pressure Ulcer Advisory Panel, European Pressure Ulcer Advisory Panel, and Stirling — are discussed. Many classification systems have been adopted by trusts despite insufficient research in their use in clinical practice. Regardless of which classification system is implemented, nurses need to be familiar with the one they are using and how to stage accurately a pressure ulcer. This can only be attained through regular education.

The use of a classification system enables accurate description of tissue damage, which gives an indication of deterioration or improvement in the patient's pressure ulcer. The practitioner assesses the skin damage and grades the skin damage in a numerical category. The aim of using a pressure classification grading system is to provide a consistent method of skin assessment using a numerical score. This promotes the passage of accurate information between the multidisciplinary team and carers on the patient's progress/deterioration (James, 1998). In addition, classification systems can aid in the decision process when considering which pressure-relieving products should be used (European Pressure Ulcer Advisory Panel [EPUAP], 1998).

Pressure ulcer grading can reflect the severity of the pressure ulcer in a number of ways by measuring the depth of the ulcer, the area of the skin affected, and the layers of skin damaged (James, 1998; National Institute for Clinical Excellence, 2001). There are a number of advantages and disadvantages for using classification systems as shown in *Table 5.1*.

Fletcher (1995) states that classification grading systems have been developed to assist nurses with gathering consistent information and defining and describing skin damage, and that they improve diagnosis, treatment and allocation of resources. Evaluating pressure ulcer data is confounded by the lack of agreement on the grading of pressure ulcers.

During the last thirty years, many classification systems for pressure ulcers have been introduced into patient care and are now in daily use. Classification systems suffer the common problems associated with risk assessment tools, ie. nurses accept the systems that they have been given to use and do not always question them. They do not stop to think whether the system has been adequately researched and validated and its reliability confirmed (Walsh and Ford, 1989). Therefore, classification systems are often incorporated by trusts into pressure ulcer guidelines despite the lack of evidence for their reliability and validity.

Table 5.1: Advantages and disadvantages of classification systems in pressure area care

Advantages	• To highlight the patients at risk of developing pressure ulcers when used alongside clinical judgment • To enable limited resources to be deployed effectively • To be able to devise a plan of care to demonstrate interventions based on the classification of a pressure ulcer to prevent further skin deterioration • To be able to measure patient outcomes and grade systems that have been developed to help assist nurses with gathering consistent information and defining and describing skin damage (a method by which point prevalence and incidence can be measured, which can enhance information when compared to previous years)
Disadvantages	• Inaccuracy by different users • Complexity of scoring systems • Difficulty in assessing the depth of skin damage, eg. subcutaneous tissues or deeper layers of the skin • Approximately sixteen different classifications of skin damage exist

Classification of pressure ulcers is, however, essential because it provides a baseline to measure the outcome of a hospital's progress year on year in the form of incidence and prevalence data. The classification allows an individual's progress to be monitored and the nursing care to be adjusted accordingly. Consequently, classification systems are widely used despite the limited evidence to support them. Where a classification system has been imposed without previous education, the information obtained from it by the staff is often inconsistent. Furthermore, the staff may not understand the pathophysiology underlying pressure ulcer development (Young, 1996).

Nurses should be familiar with their adopted classification system in order to make accurate assessment for their record keeping. The ideal method of assessment is to take a photograph, as a photograph leaves no doubt about the skin damage (Louis, 1992) (but this facility is not always available), or to trace and take manual measurements of a pressure ulcer. It is only by recording this information and evaluating the outcome that the effectiveness of the classification system can be measured.

Inaccurate staging of a wound may have more far-reaching effects than practitioners realize, such as the inappropriate use of dressings and support surfaces. If the skin damage is not detected early and preventive action taken then deep vein damage will be sustained (Arnold and Walterworth, 1995). Litigation cases have increased and the grading and documentation of the pressure ulcers provide crucial evidence as to the severity of the pressure ulcer (Tingle, 1997). However, there is no national agreement on a suitable grading system which meets the criteria of reliability and validity while being simple to use.

There are many variables to be considered when classifying pressure ulcers. This is far more complicated than it appears, as some nurses' knowledge of different layers of the skin and their ability to recognize the stage of healing of a wound is limited (Young, 1996). This lack of understanding can only be addressed by a good education programme on the classification of pressure ulcers and wound definitions.

National agreement on the classification of pressure ulcers would have positive benefits, allowing comparison between different clinical environments. Research needs to pinpoint the effectiveness of classification and use of wound care products and pressure-relieving mattresses. Once a system has been selected, it is important that appropriate training is given to the users (Fletcher, 1995). Documentation presented in a clear and legible format using diagrams and text is helpful. Training should not occur just once — follow-up sessions

Glossary

Erythema: non-specific redness, generally localized and accompanied by infection (Grey, 1998)

Reactive hyperaemia: bright red flush of the skin associated with increased bloodflow following the release of the occlusion of the circulation (Lewis and Grant, 1925; Bliss, 1998)

Blanching hyperaemia: the distinct erythema caused by reactive hyperaemia. However, the skin still blanches or whitens if light finger pressure is applied which indicates the patient's micro-circulation is intact (Bliss, 1998; Collier, 1999)

Non-blanching hyperaemia: this is indicated where there is no skin colour change of the erythema when light finger pressure is applied, indicating that the patient's microcirculation is not intact (Bliss, 1998; Collier, 1999)

should be organized, eg. mandatory updates. Classification of pressure ulcers can be monitored by regular evaluation, particularly through link nurses, when prevalence audits are undertaken on a yearly basis.

Classification of pressure ulcers

There are approximately sixteen published pressure ulcer classification systems (Healey, 1996). An area of conformity on classification scales is that the higher numbers denote the more severe grade of pressure ulcer. The description of ulcers can contrast from superficial to indurated area of swelling, heat and erythema with superficial breakdown limited to the epidermis (Shea, 1975).

A particular problem is the practitioner not being able to recognize a pressure ulcer in its early stage or identify the depth of tissue damage. Lack of clarity on how to use the grading systems may account for some nurses being unable to detect pressure ulcers in the early stage (Reid and Morison, 1994; Healey, 1996). Other variables may also be responsible, eg. friction, shear, health, mobility, age, body weight, incontinence, nutrition, and blood supply.

This chapter will discuss four classification systems — the Torrance, Stirling, National Pressure Ulcer Advisory Panel and European Pressure Ulcer Advisory Panel systems — and their history, reliability and validity. These four examples are the most commonly used classification systems.

The Torrance system

The Torrance classification grading system has been in common use for the last ten years (*Table 5.2*). However, it was not tested for its reliability before it was introduced (Torrance, 1983).

Table 5.2: The Torrance classification system	
Stage 1	Blanching hyperaemia: reactive hyperaemia causes a distinct erythema after pressure is released. Light finger pressure will cause blanching of this erythema, indicating that the micro-circulation is intact
Stage 2	Non-blanching hyperaemia: here the erythema remains when light pressure is applied, indicating a degree of microcirculatory disruption and inflammation. Oedema causes distortion and thickening of all the tissues compressed between bone and the support surface. Superficial damage may present as swelling, induration, blistering or epidermal ulceration which might expose the dermis. If sensory innervation is intact, pain will be present. Friction can cause similar injuries
Stage 3	Ulceration progresses through the dermis to its junction with subcutaneous tissue. The ulcer's edges are distinct, but it is surrounded by erythema and induration. At this stage, the damage is reversible
Stage 4	The lesion now extends into the subcutaneous fat. Small vessel thrombosis and infection compound fat necrosis. Underlying muscle is swollen and inflamed and undergoes pathological changes. The relatively avascular deep fascia temporarily impedes downwards progress but promotes lateral extension, causing undermining of the skin. Epidermal thickening creates a distinct ulcer margin but inflammation, fibrosis and retraction distort the deeper areas of the ulcer
Stage 5	Infective necrosis penetrates down to the deep fascia. Destruction of muscle now occurs rapidly. The wound spreads along fascial planes and bursae, joints and body cavities can become involved. Osteomyelitis can easily develop. Multiple ulcers may communicate, resulting in massive areas of tissue destruction

Source: Torrance, 1983

Controversy over the Torrance grading system exists as to when blanching hyperaemia becomes non-blanching hyperaemia. Some practitioners argue that blanching hyperaemia is a normal physiological activity of the body and cannot be counted as skin damage; also, the time parameters of when the skin damage becomes persistent is not known and requires further research (James, 1998).

The NHS Executive's clinical guidelines on pressure ulcer risk assessment and prevention (NHS Executive, 2001) state that blanching erythema should be classed as grade 1. Lyder (1991) states that a grade 1 pressure ulcer definition represents a skin area that is pale pink to bright red in colour and this indicates that inflammation is in progress two to five days after the initial injury. The change in skin colour has proved to be a precursor to stage 1 pressure ulcer (James, 1998).

Skin that shows blanchable erythema must be considered a precursor to stage 1 pressure ulcer. True non-blanchable skin is one of the true indicators of early damage (International Association of Enterostomal Therapy, 1988). Non-blanchable erythema indicates extensive skin damage but early intervention can sometimes reverse the damage.

The rise in skin temperature can indicate skin damage as the inflammatory process has commenced, causing increased blood supply to the area and oedema and engorgement of surrounding tissues (Boarini *et al*, 1987). Conversely, the skin may feel cool to touch in non-blanchable erythema because of decreased blood supply (Parish *et al*, 1988). Lyder (1991) states that unresolved erythema after two hours should be considered a grade 1 pressure ulcer. A grade 1 pressure ulcer may appear to have oedema or induration that is ill-defined because of the pressure that caused the skin separation and allowed interstitial fluid to escape (Long, 1986). Lyder (1991) states that the skin area with intact epidermis must also be included in a grade 1 pressure ulcer criterion.

Harker (2000) claims that there is general consensus that a grade 1 Torrance is persistent non-blanching erthyema. Grade 2 is considered to be non-blanching hyperaemia although epidermal blistering is included in this category. Hitch (1995) confuses the issue further by stating Torrance grade 2 presents as a superficial ulcer or as blisters involving the epidermis or dermis. Torrance does not account for patients with little or no subcutaneous fat, as some patients are extremely emaciated. Pressure ulcers do not always develop in a set sequence consistent with the Torrance staging. There is also no provision made for how vasculitic lesions or malignancy can be classified (Harker, 2000).

The Torrance classification system does not allow specification of deep full-thickness necrotic areas (Phillips, 1997). Deeply bruised but intact skin is also not accounted for in this classification system.

The Stirling system

The Stirling pressure ulcer severity scale aimed to achieve a classification system that is relevant for use by all nurses. It also attempted to classify pressure ulcers using a system applicable to wound care specialists and researchers who require more sophisticated wound description (Reid and Morison, 1994).

It had been agreed for a long time that a national grading system was necessary. In October 1992, in an attempt to reach an agreement, a conference was held with a panel of fourteen people at Stirling Royal Hospital. The aim of this meeting was to examine the existing systems, identify the practical problems and design an easier grading system. A tool was designed to take into account epidemiology, clinical trials, teaching and patient care settings (*Table 5.3*).

This classification gave an in-depth description of ulcers, skin tone and presence of infarction and gangrene (Reid and Morison, 1994). The Stirling scoring system attempted to overcome the problems associated with other classification systems by addressing factors such as wound bed and presence of infection; however, in attempting to do this it has made the scale more complex (James, 1998).

A grant was applied for to test the Stirling classification system but this bid was not successful. Subsequently, the reliability or validity of the system was not tested before its launch. Healey (1995) found it to be the least reliable and most difficult system to use because of the complexity of the Stirling and the digits.

The Stirling was a first attempt to identify some of the complex factors that need to be inherent in any devised tool. Clinical staff need a common description so that a pressure ulcer can be measured accurately (Reid and Morison, 1994).

Table 5.3: The Stirling pressure ulcer severity scale	
Stage 0	No clinical evidence of a pressure ulcer
0.0	Normal appearance, intact skin
0.1	Healed with scarring
0.2	Tissue damage but not assessed as a pressure ulcer
Stage 1	Discoloration of intact skin (light finger pressure applied to the site does not alter the discoloration)
1.1	Non-blanchable erythema with increased local heat
1.2	Blue/purple/black discoloration. The ulcer is at least stage 1
Stage 2	Partial-thickness skin loss or damage involving epidermis and/or dermis
2.1	Blister
2.2	Abrasion
2.3	Shallow ulcer, without undermining of adjacent tissue
2.4	Any of these with underlying blue-purpose-black discoloration or induration. The ulcer is at least stage 2
Stage 3	Full-thickness skin loss involving damage or necrosis of sub-cutaneous tissue but not extending to underlying bone, tendon or joint capsule
3.1	Crater, without undermining of adjacent tissue
3.2	Crater, with undermining
3.3	Sinus, the full extent of which is not certain
3.4	Full-thickness skin loss but wound bed covered with necrotic tissue (hard or leathery black-brown tissue or softer yellow-cream-grey slough) which masks the true extent of tissue damage. The ulcer is at least stage 3. Until debrided it is not possible to observe whether damage exceeds into muscle or involves damage to bone or supporting structures
Stage 4	Full-thickness skin loss with extensive destruction and tissue necrosis extending to underlying bone, tendon or joint capsule
4.1	Visible exposure of bone, tendon or capsule
4.2	Sinus assessed as extending to bone, tendon or capsule
Third-digit classification — for the nature of the wound bed	
x.x0	Not applicable
x.xx1	Clean, with partial epithelialization
x.x2	Clean, with or without granulation, but no obvious epithelialization
x.x3	Soft slough, cream-yellow-green in colour
x.x4	Hard or leathery black-brown necrotic (dead/avascular) tissue
Fourth-digit classification for infective complications	
x.xx0	No inflammation surrounding the wound bed
x.xx1	Inflammation surrounding the wound bed
x.xx2	Cellulitis bacteriologically confirmed

Source: Reid and Morison, 1994

National Pressure Ulcer Advisory Panel (NPUAP) classification

The NPUAP system was nationally agreed in 1989 by a panel of people in the USA and was based on previous classifications (Shea, 1975; International Association for Enterostomal Therapy, 1988) (please refer to *Table 5.5* and the European Pressure Ulcer Advisory Panel [EPUAP] system as the EPUAP system is based on the NPUAP system).

The NPUAP guidelines state that future studies should use the classification to enable consistent data collection. These guidelines were piloted by healthcare agencies using a small number of patients and subsequent modifications were made before implementation. On completion of the guidelines a conference held by the NPUAP and the Wound Ostomy and Continence Nurse Society was given federal support for the adoption of the guidelines for patients in acute long-term and homecare settings. The guidelines were adopted nationally across the USA and have been subjected to the greatest formal evaluation.

Reductions in the number of pressure ulcers and the associated cost have been reported as a result of the guidelines (eg. Hu *et al*, 1993; Clark, 2001). In a study in the USA, Xakellis *et al* (1998) demonstrated an incidence reduction of ulcers from 23.2% to 4.7% in a seventy-seven-bedded ward. However, the big reduction could not be purely the result of the guidelines as there were also organizational changes of the long-term care facility which could have contributed to the reduction. The organizational changes included pressure ulcer training for all new members of staff and an increase in the number of qualified staff.

The European Pressure Ulcer Advisory Panel (EPUAP)

The EPUAP produced a policy statement on the prevention of pressure ulcers in 1998 (EPUAP, 1998) (*Table 5.4*). This statement unveiled the management/ recommendations for maintaining and improving tissue tolerance to pressure to prevent injury. The EPUAP panel elected to adopt the NPUAP classification system because of its simplicity and it was commonly used in most healthcare settings in the USA. The difference between the EPUAP and the NPUAP systems is that in the NPUAP first stage no mention is made of darkly pigmented skin (*Table 5.5*).

Russell and Reynolds (2001) report a descriptive study using a questionnaire and twelve digital photographs classified by a consensus panel of experts using the EPUAP and Stirling systems plus digit classifications. The expert panel comprised five tissue viability specialists/clinical lecturers in tissue viability with many years collective experience. They examined the images over two hours. In general, consensus on wound grading was good with little argument. There was disagreement in only two images.

Two hundred subjects were recruited from a tissue viability society (n=50), EPUAP (n=50), five community trusts (n=50) and five acute trusts (n=50) in England and Wales. The subjects were asked for demographic details (qualifications achieved, number of years qualified, employment grade and how their knowledge of classification of pressure ulcers had been obtained). The second part of the questionnaire asked them to classify twelve digital photographs of pressure ulcers against the EPUAP and the Stirling plus digits.

The study demonstrated that there is considerable lack of consensus when pressure ulcers are graded using the Stirling plus digit grading system, and less disagreement when the EPUAP scale is used. The study demonstrates that the statistical returns from different hospital and community units cannot be considered to be directly comparable. Further, the study showed that clinical nurse specialists in tissue viability were the most keen to receive extra education, while ward nurses were happy with their current knowledge and did not believe further education on pressure ulcers as opposed to education on other clinical problems was necessary.

Table 5.4: The European Pressure Ulcer Advisory Panel policy statement
Skin condition should be documented daily and any changes should be recorded as soon as they are observed. Inspection must be documented. Initial skin assessment should take into account the following:
1. Bony prominences (sacrum, heels, hips, ankles, elbows, occiput) to identify early signs of pressure damage
2. Identify the condition of the skin — dryness, cracking, erythema, maceration, fragility, heat and induration: • every effort should be made to optimize the condition of the patient's skin   • assessments of patients with dark or tanned skin are especially difficult   • avoid excessive rubbing over bony prominences as this does not prevent pressure damage and may cause additional damage   • find the source of excess moisture as a result of incontinence, perspiration, or wound drainage and eliminate this, where possible. When moisture cannot be controlled, interventions that can assist in preventing skin damage should be used   • skin injury as a result of friction and shear forces should be minimized through correct positioning, transferring and repositioning techniques   • following assessment, nutritionally compromised individuals should have a plan of appropriate support and/or supplementation that meets individual needs and is consistent with overall goals of therapy   • as the patient's condition improves the potential for improving mobility and activity status exists. Rehabilitation efforts may be instituted if consistent with the overall goals of therapy. Maintaining activity level, mobility, and range of movement is an appropriate goal for most individuals   • all interventions and outcomes should be monitored and documented

Source: EPUAP, 1998

Reliability and validity

Most classifications systems have been adopted without large-scale trials to compare their effectiveness in clinical practice, eg. the Torrance and Stirling. This omission needs to be addressed in order to provide a classification system that practitioners can use daily, and with consistency and which has measurable outcomes. National and even European classification is essential for standardization of patient care.

There has also been little research into nurses' understanding of the classification of pressure ulcers and this requires investigation as more than half a dozen pressure ulcer grading systems are in common use (Heenan, 1994).

One study observed 109 qualified staffs' grading of photographs of pressure ulcers in Caucasian patients (Healey, 1995). Three grading classification systems were used: Stirling digit 1, Torrance and Surrey (very similar to EPUAP) (grade 1 non-blanching erythema, grade 2 superficial break in the skin, grade 3 destruction of the skin without cavity, grade 4 destruction of the skin with cavity) (David *et al*, 1983).

The sample consisted of seven trusts in North-East England. Opinions were sought on the simplicity of use for the individual grading systems. The level of agreement was demonstrated to be: Surrey 67%, Torrance 60% and the Stirling 39% (when digit 1 was used it rose to 59%). The least complex grading system was preferred by the nurses — Surrey 57%, Torrance 16% and Stirling 11%. Healey stated that photographs (of ten different examples of tissue damage, from extensive crater to local redness) were not the ideal way to carry out the survey as the quality of the photograph has to be good and the skin cannot be palpated as in a normal assessment of the skin, and that real-life observations need to be considered for further studies.

A larger number of examples of different pressure ulcers would have given a more reliable data set. The grading classifications that are less complex may be more reliable but this was not addressed in this study and further work needs to be undertaken. One reason given by the author for the results on the classification systems was because of the detail required by the complex classifications that may bewilder the assessor and lead to confusion. There was no agreement on the severity of the grades demonstrated on any of the classification systems.

Table 5.5: The European Pressure Ulcer Advisory Panel classification system*

Stage 1	Non-blanchable erythema of intact skin. This may be difficult to identify in darkly pigmented skins
Stage 2	Partial-thickness skin loss involving epidermis and/or dermis: the pressure ulcer is superficial and presents clinically as an abrasion, blister or shallow crater
Stage 3	Full-thickness skin loss involving damage or necrosis of subcutaneous tissue that may extend down to, but not through, underlying fascia: the pressure ulcer presents clinically as a deep crater with or without undermining of adjacent tissue
Stage 4	Extensive destruction tissue necrosis, or damage to muscle, bone or supporting structures with or without full-thickness skin loss

*This system is based on the National Pressure Ulcer Advisory Panel Classification (NPUAP) system. The main difference between the two systems is that the EPUAP system mentions darkly pigmented skin. Source: EPUAP, 1998

Buntinx and Becker (1995) conducted a small study on interobserver variation in assessment of skin ulcers. Three nurses and three physicians, with chronic wound experience, studied twenty-four skin ulcers using five classification systems to evaluate reliability and validity. Some of the classification systems were very complex and this meant many variables had to be observed. The adapted version of Shea's pressure classification demonstrated greater agreement between observers.

The authors state that a pressure ulcer classification should not be used when more than one person performs the assessment. Acknowledgement is made that the intraobserver reliability was not assessed. Recommendations are made that classification reliability needs to be investigated for comparability and replication of this type of study.

Montgomery-Hunter *et al* (1995) demonstrated the effectiveness of a pressure ulcer prevention and early intervention programme that reduced the prevalence of pressure ulcers in a rehabilitation setting. Forty non-acute rehabilitation patients were recruited from home or from community centres. All over the age of eighteen consented to participate in the audit over a sixteen-month period. All patients were assessed on the Braden score (Braden and Bergstrom, 1994), which had been modified for this facility and the threshold that placed the patient at risk was eighteen or lower. All pressure ulcers were assessed using the NPUAP (1989) consensus statement. Protocols were produced for both prevention and treatment interventions. Education on assessment, treatment and prevention was provided for all current staff as well as new employees.

The skin assessment tool included a definition of the pressure ulcer, description and staging and a diagram of all body parts to be assessed. The result demonstrated that a reduction in pressure ulcers (25–10%) in a sixteen-month period was achieved; however, this sample was not large enough to demonstrate statistical significance. Overall, there was a decrease of 60% in the prevalence of pressure ulcers from the baseline of 25%. Patients that did have pressure ulcers had special pressure-reducing cushions and had static overlays or low air loss mattresses at the time of skin assessment. Clearly, good documentation of skin integrity and pressure ulcer risk at the time of being admitted is essential, as is immediate implementation of measures to maintain skin integrity for those identified at risk.

Banks (1998) describes educational sessions that were held in nursing homes on classification and documentation of pressure ulcers using the Surrey, Torrance, Agency for Health Care Policy and Research (AHCPR) and Stirling grading systems. Each group consisted of four to six people, with at least one qualified nurse who was responsible for assessing the pressure ulcer damage. Ten minutes were allocated for group discussion on the definition and classification of ulcers. This was the first activity.

The second activity was to list the reasons for using a particular classification system. The third activity was to identify the potential problems that may arise. The fourth activity encouraged participants to think about pressure ulcer classification and how it relates to their setting, to compare classification systems and state why they had preference for one system and the limitations of that tool.

The conclusions do not state what the outcomes of these four activities were, but claim that staff who had attended all the first three sessions should have achieved a sound knowledge base on the development and classification of pressures ulcers.

These studies have made an attempt to answer some of the problems with classification systems and clearly more investigation is required. Large-scale trials are needed with different grades of nursing staff and consensus panels of experts for the gold standard to compare the subjects' responses. The method of assessment of pressure ulcers for research trials is problematic as photographs, while the best method, are not the most practical in terms of maintaining a patient's modesty.

Conclusion

It is essential that nurses who are assessing the patients' pressure areas have a good knowledge of the classification system being used by their establishment. Education should not just be given on a one-off basis but every one to two years. There is very little research to investigate the reliability and validity of classification systems. Some classification systems currently in use in some establishments have been adopted without validation studies, eg. Stirling and Torrance, and with little educational instruction. It appears that classification systems have been accepted on face validity and not on reliability and inter-rater reliability.

Classifications of pressure ulcers are used as measurable outcomes of patient care and therefore need to be accurate. Incidence and prevalence data also use classification of pressure ulcers and this can lead to inconsistency of information if there is insufficient training. For nurses to attain a set standard, agreement needs to be reached on a national/European classification system. This would enable the education to be standardized. Ultimately, a higher standard of patient care might be feasible with an accurate classification of pressure ulcers, giving a measurable outcome in line with today's health service culture.

Key points

⌘ A good education programme on the classification of pressure ulcers is important.

⌘ National agreement on the classification of pressure ulcers would have positive benefits, allowing comparison between different clinical environments.

⌘ Most classification systems have been adopted without large-scale trials to compare their effectiveness in clinical practice.

⌘ There has been very little research into nurses' understanding of the classification of pressure ulcers.

References

Arnold N, Walterworth B (1995) Wound staging: can nurses apply classroom education to the clinical setting? *Ostomy Wound Management* **41**(5): 40–4

Banks V (1998) The classification of pressure sores. *J Wound Care* **7**(1): 21–3

Bliss MR (1998) Hyperaemia. *J Tissue Viabil* **8**(4): 4–13

Boarini JH, Bryant RA, Zink M (1987) *Achieving Autolysis with Transparent Dressings*. 3M, Minnesota

Braden BJ, Bergstrom N (1994) Predictive validity of the Braden scale for predicting pressure ulcer risk. *Nurs Clin N Am* **22**(2): 417–28

Buntinx F, Becker H (1995) In: Cherry G, ed. Interobserver variation in the assessments of skin ulcers. 5th European Conference, Advances in Wound Management, Macmillan, London: 44–6

Clark M (2001) Pressure ulcer prevention. In: Morison M, ed. *The Prevention and Treatment of Pressure Ulcers*. Harcourt, London: 75–99

Collier M (1999) Blanching and non-blanching hyperaemia. *J Wound Care* **8**(2): 63–4

David J, Chapman RG, Chapman EG, Lockett B (1983) *An Investigation of the Current Methods Used in Nursing for the Care of Patients with Established Pressure Ulcers*. Nursing Practice Unit, Northwick Park, Middlesex

European Pressure Ulcer Advisory Panel (1998) A policy statement on prevention of pressure ulcers from the European Pressure Ulcer Advisory Panel. *Br J Nurs* **7**(15): 888–90

Fletcher J (1995) *Pressure Sore Grading*. Journal of Wound Care Resource File, Macmillan Magazines, London

Fletcher J (1997) Pressure sore treatment. *J Wound Care* **6**(8): 398–400

Grey J (1998) Cellulitis associated with wounds. *J Wound Care* **7**(7): 338–9

Harker J (2000) Pressure ulcer classification: the Torrance system. *J Wound Care* **9**(6): 275–7

Healey F (1995) The reliability and utility of pressure sore grading systems. *J Tissue Viabil* **5**(4): 111–14

Healey F (1996) Classification of pressure sores: 2. *Br J Nurs* **5**(9): 567–74

Heenan A (1994) Hobson's choice. *J Wound Care* **3**(2): 59

Hitch S (1995) NHS Executive Nursing Directorate strategy for major clinical guidelines: prevention and management of pressure sores: a literature review. *J Tissue Viabil* **5**(1): 3–11

Hu TW, Scotts NA, Fogarty TE, Bergstrom N (1993) Cost analysis for guideline implementation in prevention and early treatment of pressure ulcers. *Decubitus* **6**(2): 42–6

International Association for Enterostomal Therapy (1988) Dermal wounds: pressure sores. Philosophy of the IAET. *J Enterostomal Ther* **15**: 4–17

James HM (1998) Classification and grading of pressure sores. *Prof Nurse* **13**(10): 669–72

Lewis T, Grant R (1925) Observations upon reactive hyperaemia in man. *Heart* **12**: 73–120

Long RL (1986) Current concepts in clinical therapeutics: pressure sores. *Clin Pharm* **5**: 669–81

Louis DT (1992) Photographing pressure ulcers to enhance documentation. *Decubitus* **5**(4): 44–5

Lyder CH (1991) Conceptualization of stage 1 pressure ulcer. *J ET Nurs* **18**(5): 162–5

Montgomery-Hunter S, Langemo DK, Olson B *et al* (1995) The effectiveness of skin care protocols for pressure ulcers. *Rehabil Nurs* **20**(5): 250–5

National Institute for Clinical Excellence (2001) *Pressure Ulcer Risk Assessment and Prevention*. NICE, London

NHS Executive (2001) *Clinical Practice Guidelines on Prevention and Management of Pressure Sores*. NHS Executive, Leeds

National Pressure Ulcer Advisory Panel (1989) Incidence, economics and risk assessment. *Care Sci Pract* **7**(4): 96–9

Parish LC, Witkowski JA, Crissey JT (1988) Unusual aspects of decubitus ulcers. *Decubitus* **1**: 22–4

Phillips J (1997) *Pressure Sores*. Churchill Livingstone, London

Reid J, Morison M (1994) Towards a consensus: classification of pressure sores. *J Wound Care* **3**(3): 157–60

Russell LJ, Reynolds T (2001) How accurate are pressure ulcer grades: an image-based survey of nurses' performance? *J Tissue Viabil* **11**(2): 67–75

Shea JD (1975) Pressure sores, classification and management. *Clin Orthop* **112**: 89–100

Tingle J (1997) Pressure: counting the legal cost of nursing neglect. *Br J Nurs* **6**(13): 757

Torrance C (1983) *Pressure Scores: Aetiology, treatment and prevention*. Croom Helm, Beckenham, Kent

Walsh M, Ford P (1989) Nursing rituals. In: Clay T, ed. *Pressure Sores*. Heinemann Nursing, Heinemann Professional Publishing, Oxford: 70–82

Young T (1996) Classification of pressure sores: 1. *Br J Nurs* **5**(7): 438–46

Xakellis GC, Frantz RA, Lewis A, Harvey P (1998) Cost-effectiveness of an intensive pressure ulcer prevention protocol in long-term care. *Adv Wound Care* **11**(1): 22–9

6

Lymphoedema: Components and function of the lymphatic system

Jane Board, Wendy Harlow

Lymphoedema is an incurable and debilitating condition which has a negative impact on the quality of life of the sufferer and his/her family. Information with regards to diagnosis and treatment is often scarce and conflicting in nature. The following chapter should enable nurses to recognize the condition, provide basic information to a patient and instigate treatment through referral. It describes the anatomy, physiology and functions of the lymphatic system. The focus is on the parts of the lymphatic system which are specific to the condition of lymphoedema.

The lymphatic system plays a major role in tissue fluid dynamics by transporting a fluid called lymph from the tissues to the blood circulatory system. The aim of the first section of this chapter is to describe the anatomical structures that allow the transportation of lymph and the principles of fluid exchange that enable its formation and drainage. This section also aims to help nurses understand how, as a result of a failure in the transporting capacity of the system, lymph accumulates within the tissues resulting in the condition lymphoedema.

Anatomy of the lymphatic system

The lymphatic system is made up of a fluid called lymph which flows through lymphatic vessels, nodes, ducts and organs containing lymphatic tissue (Tortora and Grabowski, 1993). Fluid (lymph) is drained from the interstitial spaces into lymphatic (initial) capillaries, which are situated in the superficial layer of the dermis. Lymphatic capillaries then fuse to form pre-collector vessels which transport the lymph through the dermal and subcutaneous layers into larger lymphatic vessels known as collectors.

At intervals along the collectors, lymph flows through lymphatic tissue structures, called lymph nodes, sometimes referred to as lymph glands. The collectors at the outlet of the nodes pass lymph on to other nodes of the same group and eventually unite to form lymph trunks. The principal trunks consolidate and pass the lymph upwards to two main channels — the thoracic duct and the right lymphatic duct.

The thoracic duct runs alongside the inferior vena cava and drains lymph into the venous system at the junction of the left internal jugular and the left sub-clavian veins. The right lymphatic duct, situated by the jugulosubclavian junction, drains lymph into the right internal jugular, subclavian and brachiocephalic veins.

In the skin, lymphatic vessels generally follow the route of veins. In the viscera, the vessels generally follow arteries (*Figure 6.1*).

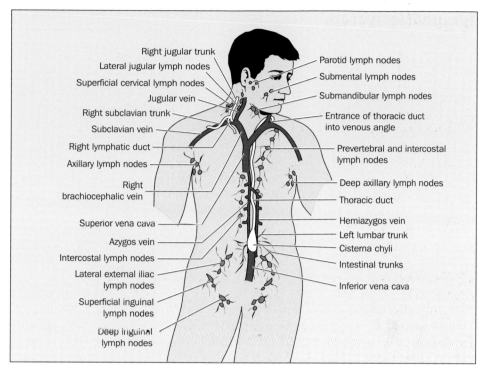

Figure 6.1: The main lymphatic pathways
© Robert Twycross (2000) *Lymphoedema*. Radcliffe Medical Press, Oxford.
Reproduced with the kind permission of the copyright holder

Part 1: Components of the lymphatic system

Lymph

Lymph is interstitial fluid that enters the lymphatic system. It is a clear or straw-coloured fluid deriving its name from the latin word lympha, which means clear water. Lymph is made up of water, macromolecules (particularly proteins), dying cells and other waste products such as urea (*Table 6.1*).

Lymphatic capillaries

Lymphatic capillaries are the most peripheral vessels and are often referred to as the initial lymphatic vessels. They are located in the superficial layer of the dermis in the extracellular tissue spaces. Lymphatic capillaries are blind-ended tubes and, unlike any other blood or lymphatic vessel, consist solely of endothelium (Mortimer, 1990). The lacteals are specialized lymphatic capillaries that extend into the intestinal villi. Their function is to absorb fat from the small intestine.

At right angles to the capillaries are structures called anchoring filaments, a delicate reticular system that attaches the endothelial cells of the capillary to the surrounding tissues (Tortora and Grabowski, 1993). Anchoring filaments provide the port of entry for interstitial fluid to enter a lymphatic capillary.

Table 6.1: Components of the lymphatic system
The lymphatic system comprises:
•   lymph
•   lymphatic capillaries
•   pre-collector vessels
•   collector vessels
•   nodes
•   lymphatic trunks
•   ducts

Pre-collector vessels

These are made up of attenuated epithelium and share a close resemblance with the capillaries. Pre-collectors commence in the mid aspect of the dermis. Valves and smooth muscle become evident as the vessels progress into the lower aspects of the dermis (Ryan, 1989). The presence of valves ensures the flow of lymph is in one direction. The function of pre-collector vessels is to propel lymph from the mid and lower aspects of the dermis into the collector vessels that are situated in the subcutaneous tissues.

Collectors, lymphatic trunks and lymphatic ducts

These are similar in structure to veins although their walls are thinner and contain more valves. Each section between valves is referred to as a lymphangion. The vessels increase in diameter and become fewer in number as they progress towards the ducts, travelling from the dermis, progressing deep into the subcutaneous tissue (Jenns and Williams, 1994). Collector vessels transport lymph through lymph nodes, uniting as lymphatic trunks, that in turn drain lymph into the venous system via the lymphatic ducts (*Figure 6.2*).

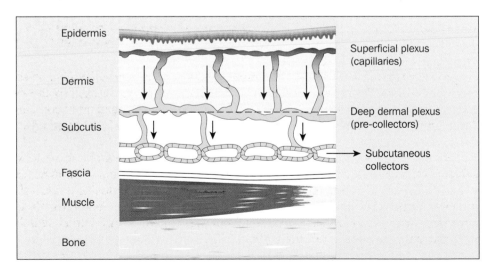

Figure 6.2: Skin and subcutaneous lymphatic vessels. This diagram is reprinted by kind permission of Churchill Livingstone, Edinburgh. Source: Mortimer, 1990

The structural layers of a lymphatic vessel

The structural layers of a lymphatic vessel are: outer layer of fibrous tissue; middle layer of muscular and elastic tissue; inner layer composed of a single layer of endothelial cells; and valves.

Lymph nodes

There are approximately 600 lymph nodes scattered throughout the body. Some nodes, such as the axillary nodes, are situated deep within the tissues; others, such as the inguinal nodes, are more superficial. Nodes may be grouped together, forming multiple nodular patches, such as the tonsils. Other nodes, eg. the urogenital nodes, exist individually.

Lymph nodes can vary considerably in size, some are as small as a pin head, others as large as an almond. They vary from 1mm to 25mm in length. Lymph nodes are covered by a capsule of fibrous tissue which dips down into the node substance forming partitions known as trabeculae. Each lymph node has three regions, the cortex, paracortex and medulla (*Figure 6.3*). The cortex or outer region is made up of densely packed lymphocytes arranged in masses and referred to as lymphatic nodules.

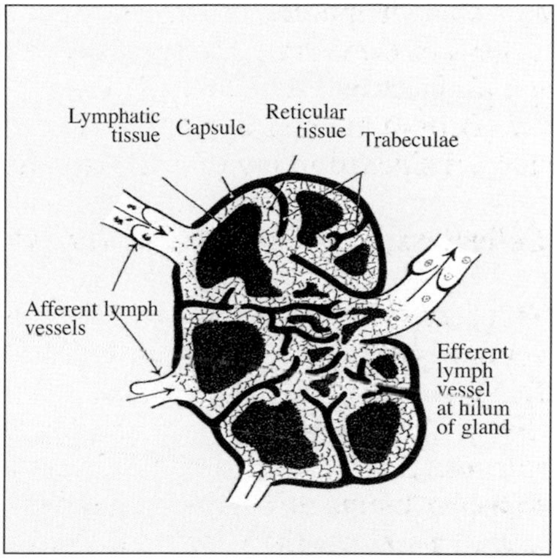

A lymphocyte is a type of white blood cell that is formed in lymphoid tissue. There are two types of lymphocytes: T-lymphocytes and B-lymphocytes. Their function is to produce immune bodies to overcome

Figure 6.3: A lymph node, showing the direction of flow of lymph.
This diagram is reprinted by kind permission of Churchill Livingstone, Edinburgh. Source: Wilson and Waugh, 1996

and protect against infection. The outer rim of the nodule contains T-lymphocytes, often referred to as T-cells and macrophages. The inner rim of the cortex, also known as the germinal centre, contains B-lymphocytes or B-cells. The paracortex contains T-cells and the medulla or inner region contains both T- and B-lymphocytes arranged into strands or chords (Bannister *et al*, 1995).

Lymph enters a node through as many as four afferent lymphatic vessels. Valves within the vessels ensure that lymph flows in one direction through the node. Having penetrated the capsule, lymph enters the cortex and medulla through a series of channels called sinuses. The lymph exits the node through no more than two efferent vessels emerging from the hilus or hilum. Blood vessels enter and leave the node at this point (*Table 6.2*).

The lymphatic ducts

Two lymphatic ducts receive lymph from the whole body and return it to the bloodstream. They are the thoracic and right lymphatic ducts. The thoracic duct commences at the cisterna chyli, a sac-like dilation on the lymphatic pathway in front of the first and second lumbar vertebrae and to the right of the abdominal aorta (Bannister *et al*, 1995). It is the largest lymphatic vessel in the body and is the main receiving duct for the lymphatic system (*Table 6.3*).

The thoracic duct contains several valves and is approximately 40cm long. This duct conveys all lymph from the lower limbs, pelvic and abdominal cavities, left side of the chest, head, neck and left arm. It then drains into the left subclavian vein. The right lymphatic duct is much shorter at approximately 1.25cm in length. It lies at the root of the neck and conveys lymph from the right side of the chest, head, neck and right arm to the right subclavian vein.

Table 6.2: Area of body drainage of lymph nodes

Major node	Area of body drainage
Axillary	Arms, thoracic wall, breast, upper abdominal wall
Supratrochlear	Hands, forearm
Cervical	Scalp, face, neck, nasal cavity, pharynx
Tracheobrachial and intercostal	Thoracic cavity
Intestinal	Abdominal viscera
Inguinal	Legs, genitalia, lower abdominal wall
Iliac	Pelvic viscera

Table 6.3: Principal lymphatic trunks, the source of drainage and the duct into which each trunk drains

Trunk	Source of drainage	Receiving duct
Lumbar (right and left)	Lower extremities, viscera of pelvis, kidneys, adrenal and abdominal wall	Thoracic
Intestinal (right and left)	Stomach, intestines, pancreas, spleen and part of the liver	Thoracic
Bronchomediastinal		
Right	Right sides of thorax, right lung, right side heart, part of liver	Right lymphatic
Left	Left side thoracic wall, anterior diaphragm, upper abdominal wall, left lung, left side heart	Thoracic
Subclavian		
Right	Right upper extremities	Right lymphatic
Left	Left upper extremities	Thoracic
Jugular		
Right	Right sides of head and neck	Right lymphatic
Left	Left sides of head and neck	Thoracic

Physiology of lymphatic system

Examination of the structure of the lymphatic system has demonstrated its ability to provide a one-way drainage system that transports lymph from the tissues to the blood circulatory system. This section will identify the mechanisms that control tissue fluid production, which enables the removal of excess interstitial fluid and the formation and drainage of lymph.

Tissue fluid dynamics

The interstitial compartment of the tissues of the body is the space outside the capillaries and between the cells (Stanton, 2000). Most components of blood plasma, with the exception of large protein molecules, flow freely through the arterial end of the capillary wall to form interstitial fluid that bathes the cells with nutrients.

Interstitial fluid is either reabsorbed back into the bloodstream at the venous end of the capillaries or drained into the lymphatic system. Approximately 16–18 litres of interstitial fluid is formed each day, a majority of which (14–16 litres) returns directly to the bloodstream. The remaining 2–4 litres is drained as lymph into the lymphatic system, consisting of water, small molecules of protein, electrolytes, fats and cell debris. Small molecules of protein are unable to return directly to the bloodstream because of the forces present within the capillaries. Therefore, interstitial fluid is continually produced and drained away (Stanton, 2000).

The mechanism that controls the exchange of fluid between interstitial fluid and blood plasma centres around the forces of filtration and reabsorption and is referred to as Starling's Law of the Capillaries (Levick, 1991a) (*Figure 6.4*). Hydrostatic and osmotic pressures are responsible for maintaining the equilibrium of fluid exchange. The hydrostatic pressure is the pressure of water in the fluid and the osmotic pressure relates to the force exerted by the plasma proteins.

To summarize, in normal health the balance between these forces is almost equal, ensuring the circulatory volume of plasma is maintained and the tissues are not congested with fluid. Thus, homeostasis, the normal standard state of the environment, is maintained within the tissues. The amount of fluid in the interstitial space at any one time is dependent upon the amount of fluid entering it (net capillary filtration rate) and the amount of fluid leaving via the venous and lymphatic systems (*Figure 6.5*).

The formation of lymph (*Figure 6.6*)

Interstitial tissues swell as they absorb the fluid which escapes from the capillaries. The effect of the rising osmotic and hydrostatic pressure pulls on the anchoring filaments of the lymphatic capillaries thereby enlarging the openings of the endothelial cells. The interstitial fluid enters the capillary and becomes known as lymph (Vander *et al*, 1990). This process enables small amounts of interstitial fluid to continually enter the lymphatic capillaries and, in so doing, prevent the accumulation of fluid in the interstitial spaces (Mortimer, 1995).

The composition of lymph and interstitial fluid is almost the same at this point, the major difference being location. The protein content of lymph is generally lower than that of plasma. In plasma, the protein concentration measures approximately 7g/dl; in lymph it measures 2.5g/dl. However, the protein content of lymph can vary within the body depending on the region being drained. For example, 2g/dl of protein is present within the skeletal muscle, 4.1g/dl within the gastrointestinal tract and as much as 6g/dl of protein concentration within the lymph drainage system of the liver (Emslie-Smith *et al*, 1988). Lymph drained from the lacteal capillaries is unique in its milky appearance because of the presence of fat droplets and is known as chyle (Levick, 1991b).

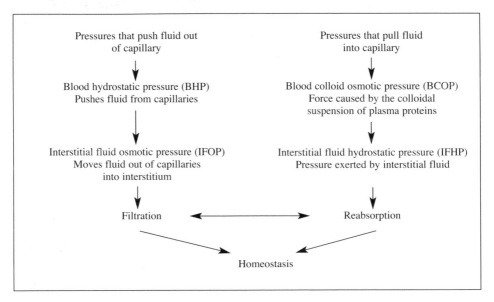

Figure 6.4: The pressure of Starling's law of the Capillaries (Levick, 1991a)

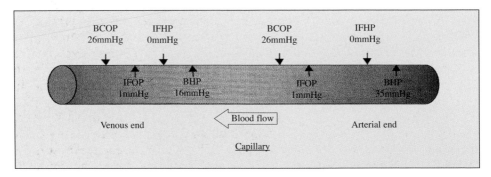

Figure 6.5: The dynamics of capillary exchange. BCOP = blood colloid osmotic pressure; IFHP = interstitial fluid hydrostatic pressure; IFOP = interstitial fluid osmotic pressure; BHP = blood hydrostatic pressure

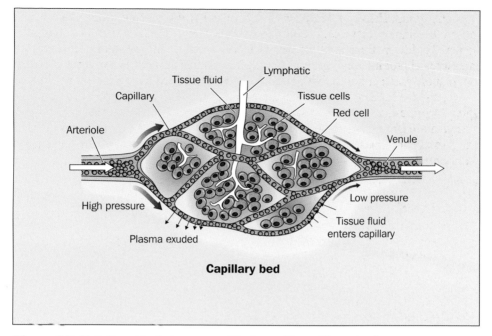

Figure 6.6: Relationship between capillaries, cells and lymphatics.
Reproduced by kind permission of John Murray, London. Source: Mackean, 1973

The filtering of lymph

Lymph is propelled into the pre-collectors and on to the larger lymphatic vessels where the lymph passes through strategically placed lymph nodes. The function of the nodes is to remove foreign substances (antigens) and prevent them entering the bloodstream. The antigens are filtered out of the lymph and become trapped within the reticular fibres of the node. The process of filtration enables the removal of foreign substances such as bacteria, phagocytes and tumour cells.

Macrophages are released to destroy the antigens by the process of phagocytosis. Alternatively, T-lymphocytes are activated to destroy other noxious material such as cancerous cells by releasing cytotoxic secretions such as interleukin and interferon. After the commencement of an immune response, B-lymphocytes proliferate into antibody-secreting plasma cells and circulate the body in response to antigens situated elsewhere (Tortora and Grabowski, 1993).

The lymph is drained from the node through the efferent vessel. The composition of the fluid has now changed because of the filtering ability of the node to remove water (Emslie-Smith *et al*, 1988). As a consequence, post-nodal lymph has a higher protein concentration and smaller volume than pre-nodal lymph (Stanton, 2000). The lymph continues its journey upwards, through the lymphatic trunks, into the cisterna chyli and finally into the thoracic duct before returning to the bloodstream.

Means of lymph propulsion

Unlike the circulatory system, lymph drainage has no extrinsic pump (heart) as a means of propulsion. The system relies on intrinsic factors for transportation of fluid from the tissue spaces to the blood circulatory system:

❖ Changes in pressure within the tissues, mainly filtration pressure, propels lymph into the lymphatic capillaries.

❖ The presence of smooth muscle in the larger vessels enables them to contract, pushing lymph in the direction dictated by the valves. As a section of a vessel (lymphangion) is filled with lymph it becomes distended and pushes the fluid through the valves and into the next lymphangion. This caterpillar-like effect is a continuous process, with lymphangions filling, contracting and pushing the lymph into the next section. Contraction of these vessels is determined mainly by the supply of lymph from the smaller vessels (Mortimer, 1995).

❖ The pulsation of neighbouring arteries compresses adjacent lymphatic vessels, assisting the flow of lymph into them.

❖ Skeletal muscle contractions compress lymph vessels, forcing lymph towards the subclavian veins (Tortora and Grabowski, 1993).

❖ Respiratory movements create a pressure gradient between the two ends of the lymphatic system. With each inhalation a negative pressure is exerted from the thoracic area which pulls fluid from the abdominal region, where the pressure is higher, towards the heart.

Conclusion

This section has identified the important role the lymphatic system plays in tissue fluid dynamics. Homeostasis is dependent on the ability of the lymphatic system to drain water, protein and other products from the tissues, returning them to the blood circulatory system in the form of lymph. Failure in the transporting capacity of the system to perform this function results in the accumulation of water and proteins within the tissues, a condition known as lymphoedema.

The next section of this chapter will describe the different types of lymphoedema and the signs and symptoms associated with the condition.

References

Bannister LH, Berry MM, Collins P, Dyson M, Dussek JE, Ferguson MWJ, eds (1995) Cardiovascular: the anatomical basis of medicine and surgery. In: *Gray's Anatomy*. 38th edn. Churchill Livingstone, Edinburgh: 1605–26

Emslie-Smith D, Paterson C, Scratcherd T, Read N, eds (1988) The body fluids. In: *Textbook of Physiology*. 11th edn. Churchill Livingstone, Edinburgh: 16–22

Jenns K, Williams A (1994) *Unpublished Notes — Lymphoedema Foundation Study Day*. Sir Michael Sobell House, Churchill Hospital, Oxford: 2–5

Levick JR (1991a) Starling's principle of fluid exchange. In: *Introduction to Cardiovascular Physiology*. Butterworth, London: 143–4

Levick JR (1991b) Circulation of fluid between plasma, interstitium and lymph. In: *Introduction to Cardiovascular Physiology*. Butterworth, London: 161–2

Mackean D (1973) Blood, its composition, function and circulation. In: *Introduction to Biology*. John Murray, London: 99

Mortimer PS (1990) Lymphatics. In: Champion RH, Pye RJ, eds. *Recent Advances in Dermatology*. Churchill Livingstone, Edinburgh: 175–92

Mortimer PS (1995) Managing lymphoedema. *Clin Exp Dermatol* **20**: 98–106

Ryan TJ (1989) Structure and function of lymphatics. *J Invest Dermatol* **93**: 218–24

Stanton A (2000) How does tissue swelling occur? The physiology and pathophysiology of interstitial fluid formation. In: Twycross R, Jenns K, Todd J, eds. *Lymphoedema*. Radcliffe Medical Press, Oxford: 11–21

Tortora GJ, Grabowski SR, eds (1993) The lymphatic system. In: *Principles of Anatomy and Physiology*. 7th edn. Harper Collins, New York: 683–9

Twycross R, Jenns K, Todd J, eds (2000) The main lymphatic pathways. In: *Lymphoedema*. Radcliffe Medical Press, Oxford

Vander A, Sherman J, Luciano D (1990) Circulation. In: *Human Physiology — The Mechanisms of Body Function*. 5th edn. MacGraw-Hill Publishing, New York: 394–6

Wilson KJW, Waugh A (1996) The lymphatic system. In: *Ross and Wilson Anatomy and Physiology — Health Issues*. 8th edn. Churchill Livingstone, Edinburgh: 42

Key points

⌘ A major function of the lymphatic system is the transportation of lymph from the tissues to the bloodstream. It plays a crucial role in the regulation of homeostasis.

⌘ Lymph flows through a series of vessels and nodes before returning to the venous circulation.

⌘ Lymph comprises water, macromolecules (particularly proteins), dying cells and other waste products.

⌘ Lymph is almost equal in composition to plasma when initially drained into the lymphatic system.

⌘ The filtering ability of the nodes changes the composition of lymph as it progresses through the system.

⌘ The lymphatic system does not possess an intrinsic pump, relying on other factors to propel lymph through the vessels; 10–20% of interstitial fluid duced each day returns to the bloodstream via the lymphatic system.

Part II: Classification, signs, symptoms and diagnosis of lymphoedema

The second section in this chapter describes the different types of lymphoedema and the signs and symptoms associated with the condition. In the preceding section, we examined the anatomy, physiology and functions of the lymphatic system in relation to the condition of lymphoedema, and demonstrated how, by acting as a one-way drainage system, the lymphatics maintain tissue homeostasis through the removal of excess fluid from the interstitial spaces. Failure or dysfunction of the system can result in lymphoedema, a condition characterized by the accumulation of fluid in the soft tissues. Lymphoedema is classified into two main groups — primary and secondary. Defining the causative factors and pathogenesis of both conditions and other forms of chronic oedema will assist the reader in the clarification of the condition. The chapter concludes with an overview of assessment criteria for diagnosis, which should assist all healthcare professionals in appropriate referral.

Lymphoedema is a swelling resulting from the excess accumulation of fluid in the tissues and is caused by inadequate lymph drainage (British Lymphology Society [BLS], 2001). It is classified into primary and secondary forms and can affect upper and lower limbs, trunk, genitalia and the head. Most cases of lymphoedema are commonly seen in the arm or leg because of the limited drainage routes from these areas (BLS, 1999).

Before exploring the pathophysiology of lymphoedema it is helpful to consider tissue fluid production and drainage in a normal lymphatic system, as described in detail in the first section of this chapter.

Tissue fluid dynamics

Starling's law of the capillaries describes the mechanism that regulates interstitial fluid exchange (Tortora and Grabowski, 1993). The principal forces involved are filtration and reabsorption and, in normal health, the balance between these two forces is almost equal. Filtration enables the fluid to enter the interstitial space from the arterial end of a capillary. Fluid leaves via the venous or lymphatic system by the process of reabsorption. Approximately 80–90% of fluid leaving the arterial end of capillaries is reabsorbed back into the blood circulation via the venous ends (Bannister *et al*, 1995). The 10–20% of remaining (excess) interstitial fluid is transported back to the blood circulation by the lymphatic system in the form of lymph (Ganong, 1995) (*Figure 6.7*).

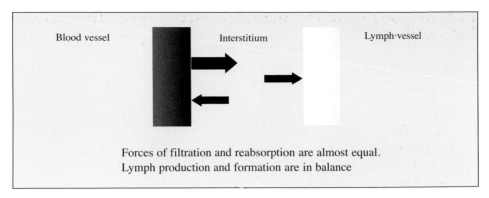

Figure 6.7: Homeostasis maintained by the lymphatics in normal health

What is oedema?

Oedema is the collection of fluid in the interstitial tissues that develops from an imbalance between the forces of filtration and reabsorption (Tortora and Grabowski, 1993). Oedema may be acute or chronic in nature. Acute oedemas occur suddenly and will resolve over a short period of time as part of the healing process, such as a sprained ankle. Chronic oedema represents a swelling that has been present for at least three months (Jenns, 2000) and is associated with conditions such as heart failure, nephrosis and cirrhosis.

Pathophysiology of the different types of chronic oedema

Lymphoedema

True lymphoedema is indicated when the principal fault lies within the lymphatic system itself (Williams, 1997). An absence, obliteration or obstruction of the lymphatic vessels affects the transporting capacity of the system (Mortimer, 1990). Lymph, which is rich in protein and other macromolecules, continues to be produced, but a dysfunction within the transporting pathway of the lymphatic vessels prevents its drainage. The problem is further compounded by the accumulation of water as a consequence of the osmotic effect of the trapped protein (Levick, 1991).

This phenomenon is characterized by a decreased rate of lymph absorption, or low-output failure of the lymph circulation (Keeley, 2000) (*Figure 6.8*). The protein content of the oedema is classed as high. However, there is a growing body of evidence that suggests the protein content could be lower than currently thought. Stanton (2000) argues that the content of oedema fluid (accumulating as a result of lymphatic drainage impairment) is almost equal to that of interstitial fluid.

Other chronic oedemas result from various combinations of lymphatic and venous insufficiency (Mortimer, 1990).

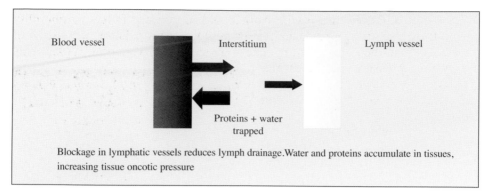

Figure 6.8: Low output failure of the lymph circulation in lymphoedema

Lymphovenous oedema

Lymphovenous oedema usually occurs as a consequence of venous disease (Mortimer, 1990). Poor venous return creates hypertension within the venous end of the capillary. A raised venous pressure increases the capillary filtration rate of water and, to a lesser extent, protein and other macromolecules into the tissues. The lymphatic system initially copes, but fails over a period of time to drain the extra load (Barrett, 1997). Consequently, fluid accumulates in the tissues, resulting in oedema. This type of oedema is described as having a high-output failure with a low protein content (Keeley, 2000) (*Figure 6.9*).

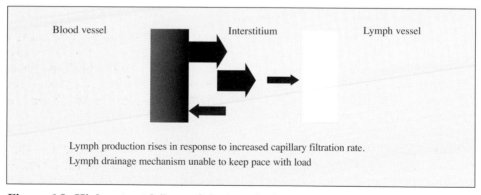

Figure 6.9: High output failure of the lymph circulation in lymphovenous oedema

Dependency/gravitational oedema

Muscle pump activity is crucial for the propulsion of blood through the venous circulation, and lymph through lymphatic vessels. Oedema can occur when a limb is dependent or immobile, and is often seen in the lower limbs in such cases as motor neurone disease, cerebral vascular accident and other forms of paralysis. It is also seen in patients who sit in a chair for long periods during the day and night, eg. those with cardiac and respiratory failure. Immobility prevents the use of the muscle and, in the absence of propulsion, congestion of blood occurs in the veins creating venous hypertension (Cameron, 1995). This backwards pressure increases the capillary filtration rate, resulting in the accumulation of fluid in the interstitium.

Lymph is also reliant on local tissue movement to propel it through the lymphatic vessels situated in the subcutaneous tissues (Mortimer, 1990). In the absence of this movement, lymph accumulates in the interstitial spaces already congested by the effects of venous hypertension.

Table 6.4 identifies the physiological effects that can occur as a consequence of a failure in lymph drainage.

Table 6.4: Consequences of lymph drainage failure	
Lymph drainage fails is	Insufficient number of transport vessels
	Insufficient forces generated to prompt drainage
	Obstruction of drainage pathways
	Increased production of lymph (mixed aetiology)
Causing	Overload of lymphatic vessels
	Reduced contractility
	Build-up of lymph in tissues and vessels
	Osmotic retention of water

Types of lymphoedema

Primary lymphoedema

Primary lymphoedema has no identifiable cause and is assumed to be caused by an intrinsic defect of the lymphatic pathways (BLS, 2001) (*Figure 6.10*). There can be either a complete absence (Williams, 1997) or hypoplasia (underdevelopment) of vessels (Mortimer, 1995a). Primary lymphoedema can affect one or more limbs and can develop at various stages of life. It can be classified into the following forms (BLS, 2001):

Milroy's disease: This describes a congenital, familial lymphoedema that results from a mutation of the gene for vascular endothelial growth factor 3. Mutation of the gene is responsible for the abnormal development of lymphatic vessels (BLS, 2001). The term Milroy's disease is often used loosely to describe a variety of different types of primary lymphoedema, producing a diagnosis that is not always strictly correct. In the future, a better understanding of the genetics involved is likely to aid diagnosis and refine the classification of this form of lymphoedema (Keeley, 2000).

Lymphoedema congenita: This form is present at or soon after birth.

Lymphoedema praecox: This develops before thirty-five years of age.

Lymphoedema tarda: This form develops after thirty-five years of age.

Secondary lymphoedema

Secondary lymphoedema can result from a variety of different extrinsic factors, each causing a disruption in the lymphatic flow. The ability of the lymphatic channels to propel the lymph forward becomes impaired, and fluid accumulates in the tissues and vessels (Wilson and Bilodeau, 1989). The causes of secondary lymphoedema are listed below.

Filariasis: Filariasis is the main cause of secondary lymphoedema world-wide, occurring as a consequence of direct parasitic invasion into the lymphatic system (Wilson and Bilodeau, 1989). The filarial larva is deposited by the mosquito into lymphatic channels where it develops into an adult worm. Filariasis is estimated to affect more than 120 million people world-wide (World Health Organization, 2001).

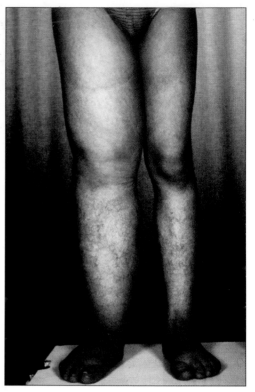

Figure 6.10: Primary lymphoedema of the right leg. No identifiable cause known, assumed to be an intrinsic defect of lymphatic pathways

Tumour: The presence of a malignancy obstructs the lymphatic drainage channels.

Surgery: The surgical removal of lymph nodes (adenectomy) disrupts lymphatic pathways.

Radiation: The process of radiotherapy is known to destroy cancerous cells and healthy tissue, including lymphatics. The fibrotic tissue that develops as a consequence of treatment prevents the regeneration of lymphatic channels and is often referred to as radiation fibrosis (Kirshbaum, 2000) *(Figure 6.11)*.

Infection/inflammation: The presence of stagnant, protein-rich oedema in the tissues predisposes to low-grade infection or inflammation (Jeffs, 1993).

Trauma: Secondary lymphoedema as a result of trauma, such as road traffic accidents and burns, is caused by the destruction of tissue.

The development of lympho-edema

The onset of lymphoedema cannot be predicted. Developments in genetic research may increase the predictive ability we have in the future, especially in primary lymphoedemas with familial history. In secondary lymphoedema of an obstructive nature, the pathogenesis of the condition is well documented. However, certain characteristics in the development and progression of the condition highlight the possible existence of underlying pathophysiological mechanisms and risk factors that may precipitate secondary lymphoedema of an obstructive nature. Characteristics include:

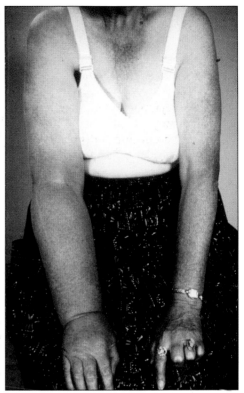

Figure 6.11: Secondary lymphoedema of the right arm. Oedema has occurred as a consequence of radiotherapy to the axilla following a mastectomy to eliminate cancer

- onset of lymphoedema not following a defined pattern of development
- latent periods between cancer/cancer treatment and onset of swelling vary from months to years in different individuals (Mortimer *et al*, 1996)
- swelling is often rapid in onset and then slow to progress
- variation in the quality of tissue swelling between patients. Some swellings are pitting, some are brawny and others are fatty in consistency (Stanton, 2000).

Health professionals and patients are known to attribute several aspects of cancer/cancer treatment to the onset of limb swelling. These include:

- histology
- type of surgical procedure
- wound drainage, wound complications and treatment
- venepuncture in the ipsilateral limb
- exercise and range of movement in the limb.

There is also some evidence that age and weight may be factors relating to the onset of the condition (Pezner, 1986; Tadych, 1987). The evidence base is currently weak in this area. Ongoing research and developments in technology, such as lymphatic imaging, continually add to the body of knowledge in lymphoedema morbidity related to cancer and its treatment.

Signs and symptoms of lymphoedema

Patients with lymphoedema can suffer from a wide range of physical, psychological and social problems as a result of their condition (Bianchi and Todd, 2000).

Physical symptoms

The presence and severity of signs and symptoms will depend on the type and duration of oedema and the history of treatment. In the early stages all forms of chronic oedema present with reversible, pitting oedema that disappears spontaneously after a night of rest (Daroczy *et al*, 1996). Venous-related oedemas, with a high water, low protein content, tend to be soft and exhibit an easy displacement of tissue fluid on pressure.

Lymphoedema that is rich in protein will, if left untreated, present with swelling that is irreversible and non-pitting, together with tissue that is fibrotic (hardened). Over a period of time other changes to the skin may develop as a consequence of the stagnating proteins within the tissues. Untreated oedema resulting from venous insufficiency will eventually lead to lymphatic failure, with symptoms manifesting as true lymphoedema (Mortimer, 1990).

Clinical features

Oedema: Visible swelling that can affect one or more limbs and extend into the trunk of the body that is adjacent to the swollen limb.

Skin changes: These include:

* Dry skin: The skin turgor is diminished as a consequence of swelling, resulting in the epidermis becoming rough, scaly and flaky (Veitch, 1993).
* Taut/shiny skin: The effect of swelling can distend the skin to give it a taut and shiny appearance.
* Skinfolds: Folds and crevices occur in response to large amounts of oedema.
* Lymphangiomas (*Figure 6.12*): Bulging skin lymphatics on the surface of the skin resembling blisters. Usually an indication of compromised flow within the deeper lymphatic channels (Mortimer, 1995b).
* Papillomatosis (*Figure 6.13*): A cobblestone appearance of the skin caused by dilated and distended skin lymphatics surrounded by fibrotic tissue (Keeley, 2000).
* Hyperkeratosis: A warty, scaly change to the skin created by a build-up of the stratum corneum layer of the skin (BLS, 2001). The effect of skin creases, dermal turgor, papillomatosis and hyperkeratosis give the epidermis a thickened texture, sometimes referred to as elephantiasis because the skin resembles elephant hide. These symptoms are most commonly seen in the lower limbs and occur as a consequence of the long-term accumulation of protein-rich oedema.
* Acute inflammatory episodes: A condition usually characterized by

constitutional upset, erythematous rash and increased swelling (BLS, 2001). A break in the skin enables bacteria to enter and proliferate within the lymphoedematous tissue, resulting in inflammation and infection. Attacks of acute inflammatory episodes start rapidly, often without warning. The patient suddenly feels unwell. The limb becomes hot, tender and inflamed. Capillary filtration is increased in response to the inflammatory reaction, with production of further oedema (Jeffs, 1993).

❖ Unlike conventional cellulitis, there is no clearly demarcated erythema because the inflammatory process spreads rapidly throughout the oedematous tissues, usually the whole limb (Mortimer, 2001). Severe attacks can produce fever, rigours, headaches and vomiting. Treatment centres around bedrest, antibiotics and, in severe cases, hospitalization.

❖ Lymphorrhoea: This is caused by the leakage of lymph through break(s) in the skin from trauma or an exacerbation of oedema (Ling *et al*, 1997). Large, often copious amounts of fluid appear on the skin, trickling down the limb.

Subcutaneous tissue changes: Fingertip pressure on oedematous skin produces a depression lasting a few seconds, when fluid in the tissues is easily displaced (Daroczy *et al*, 1996). In the latent stages of lymphoedema, the application of pressure by the finger no longer displaces fluid because of fibrotic changes occurring in the tissues as a consequence of accumulating proteins (Levick, 1991). The pitting test is a useful tool for ascertaining the effects of oedema on the subcutaneous tissues.

Stemmer's sign (see *Figure 6.12*)*:* Thickened skin-folds prevent the pinching of thickened skin on the upperside of the toes, particularly at the base of the second toe. This is a unique test in confirming the diagnosis of lymphoedema.

Pain: Patients will use a range of adjectives to describe their pain. Some will complain of an ache or heaviness associated with the weight of their limb (Carroll and Rose, 1992); others may have pain specific to the presence of lesions from other active disease, acute inflammatory episodes or the pressure of oedema on nerve endings (Badger *et al*, 1988).

Joint immobility (*Figure 6.14*)*:* The physical weight of an oedematous limb can impair movement and function. In addition, reduced dexterity will impede upon everyday activities such as washing, combing hair and driving. Any degree of pain will further compound the restricted use of the limb.

Psychosocial factors

The impact of the lymphoedema can have far-reaching consequences, both psychologically and socially (Gillham, 1994). An oedematous limb creates different visible contours, and distress for the patient (Price, 1992). Difficulties are often encountered purchasing clothes (Bennington, 1991). The distortion in the size of one area of the body can reduce self-esteem and present problems with the perception of body image (Woods *et al*, 1995).

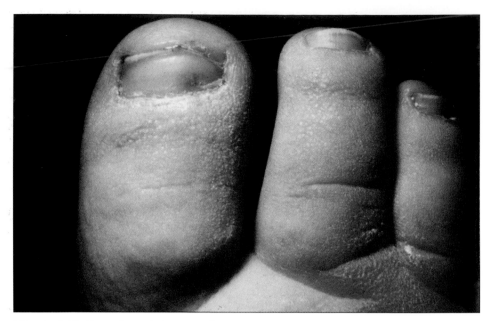

Figure 6.12: Lymphangiomas can be seen on the skin surface. Thickened skin at the base of the second toe prevents the pinching of skin, resulting in a positive Stemmers' sign.
Reproduced courtesy of Professor Peter Mortimer, Consultant Dermatologist, St George's Hospital, London

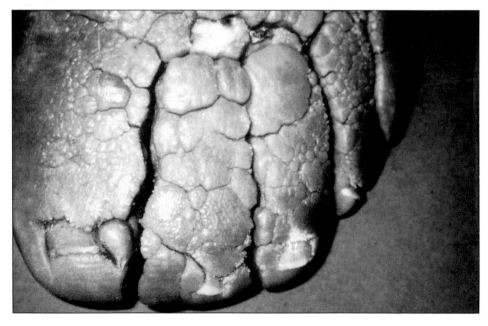

Figure 6.13: Papillomatosis: a cobblestone appearance of the skin is shown

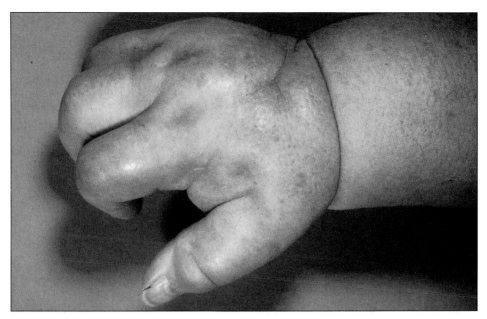

Figure 6.14: Severe oedema has reduced dexterity of the fingers and impeded functional use

An oedematous limb can also affect sexual relations with a partner, and social interactions with family and friends (Barrett, 1997). A reduction in the functional use of the limb can create stress within the home environment as other members of the family are relied upon for everyday tasks. It may also have major implications in the workplace. Addressing such issues will not only help in relieving anxiety and emotional distress, but can also enhance self-esteem and motivation to cope with the requirements of treatment.

Assessment

Clinical features and associated symptoms need to be systematically evaluated to ascertain diagnosis. This is achieved through assessment, which can:

- confirm the diagnosis of lymphoedema
- quantify the presence of clinical features
- organize a programme of treatment
- identify factors that could affect the outcome of treatment.

This is achieved by:

- obtaining a comprehensive medical history
- acquiring details of the onset and duration of the oedema, and predisposing factors
- performing a physical examination of the affected and non-affected limbs.

An accurate medical history eliminates oedemas from other causes, such as cardiac, renal and hepatic disease. Treatment of oedemas of central origin are contraindicated in this instance and should be returned to the referral source. Obtaining details of the onset, duration and predisposing factors further assists in the confirmed diagnosis of lymphoedema.

The unaffected limb provides a baseline measurement and should therefore be included in all aspects of physical examination. Subjective examination of the swollen limb reveals the site and extent of the oedema, including the trunk (Jenns, 2000). Examination of the skin and subcutaneous tissues aids diagnosis, reveals the severity of the condition and provides an indication of the treatment that is necessary (Shankar *et al*, 2000). The affected and non-affected limbs are measured to identify the total excess volume, the distribution of fluid within the limb and the degree of distortion in shape (Badger, 1993). Limb volume is calculated by recording circumferential measurements at 4cm intervals along the limb and using the cylinder formula:

$$\frac{\text{Circumference}^2}{\pi}$$

In the case of unilateral swelling, the percentage volume difference can be calculated by comparing the measurements taken from both limbs using the formula:

$$\frac{100 \text{ x excess limb volume}}{\text{normal limb volume}}$$

The degree of distortion in shape can also be calculated by dividing the measurements of the proximal (upper) segment of a limb by the distal (lower) segment of the same limb. This ratio is then compared for both limbs, and by subtracting the swollen ratio from the normal ratio, the difference is established. In cases of bilateral limb oedema, the percentage volume and distortion of shape cannot be calculated, and the matter of degree in both instances remains a subjective one.

Subjective assessment of the epidermis reveals the general condition of the skin and the presence of complications. Palpation of the skin enables the texture of the subcutaneous tissues to be examined (see 'Clinical features' — subcutaneous tissue changes).

Currently there are no validated assessment tools to quantify the severity of skin changes, although some have been developed by expert practitioners in the field (Badger and Jeffs, 1995). The assessment tools in use aim to identify the category of need through a process of scoring for presenting clinical features. A high score reflects severe skin changes requiring intensive treatment.

In summary, an assessment that is thorough and methodical in its approach enables the correct diagnosis to be established, the severity of the condition to be identified and the appropriate treatment to be instigated.

Conclusion

This section has defined the causative factors and pathogenesis of primary and secondary lymphoedema and other forms of chronic oedema. It highlights the need to understand the mechanisms of tissue fluid dynamics in normal health in order to differentiate the pathophysiological process of each type of chronic oedema. Details of a patient's medical history and the onset, duration and predisposing factors of the oedema assist with the clarification of diagnosis. The identification of clinical features, further assists with ascertaining diagnosis.

Key points

⌘ Oedema is the collection of fluid in the interstitial tissues that develops from an imbalance between the forces of filtration and reabsorption.

⌘ Lymphoedema occurs as a consequence of a failure within the transporting capacity of the lymphatic system.

⌘ Lymphoedema is classified into two main groups, primary and secondary.

⌘ The onset of lymphoedema cannot be predicted.

⌘ Filariasis is the most common cause of secondary lymphoedema.

⌘ Papillomatosis and hyperkeratosis are skin changes that are characteristic of lymphoedema.

⌘ The psychosocial effects of a patient's lymphoedema can often be overshadowed by the presence of physical symptoms.

⌘ Assessment enables the cause of the oedema to be established, the severity of the condition to be identified and the appropriate treatment to be instigated.

References

Badger C (1993) Guidelines for the calculation of limb volume based on surface measurements. British Lymphology Interest Group Newsletter, Sevenoaks, Kent **7**: 3–7

Badger C, Jeffs E (1995) Selection of treatment score: 'the five S score'. Unpublished notes, St Catherine's Hospice, Crawley

Badger CMA, Mortimer PS, Regnard CFB, Twycross RG (1988) Pain in the chronically swollen limb. In: Partsch H, ed. *Progress in Lymphology — XI*. Elsevier Science, Oxford: 234–6

Bannister LH, Berry MM, Collins P, eds (1995) Lymphatic system. In: Gray's *Anatomy: The Anatomical Basis of Medicine and Surgery*. 38th edn. Churchill Livingstone, Edinburgh: 1605–26

Barrett J (1997) The assessment and treatment of patients with lymphoedema. *Nurs Standard* **11**(21): 49–56

Bennington G (1991) Nursing management of lymphoedema. *Nurs Standard* **6**(7): 24–7

Bianchi J, Todd M (2000) The management of a patient with lymphoedema of the legs. *Nurs Standard* **14**(40): 51–6

British Lymphoedema Society (1999) *Strategy for Lymphoedema Care*. BLS, Sevenoaks, Kent

British Lymphoedema Society (2001) *Clinical Definitions*. BLS, Sevenoaks, Kent

Cameron J (1995) Venous and arterial leg ulcers. *Nurs Standard* **9**(26); 25–30

Carroll D, Rose K (1992) Treatment leads to significant improvement: effect of conservative treatment on pain in lymphoedema. *Profess Nurse* **8**(1): 32–6

Daroczy J, Schingale FJ, Mortimer PS (1996) Definition of lymphoedema. In: Kaufmann R, Weilhermuller M, eds. *Practical Ambulant Lymphology*. Varlag Medical Concept, Munchen, Germany: 15–16

Ganong WF (1995) Dynamics of blood and lymph flow. In: *Review of Medical Physiology*. 17th edn. Prentice-hall, London: 537–41

Gillham L (1994) Lymphoedema and physiotherapists: control not cure. *Physiotherapy* **80**(12): 835–43

Jeffs E (1993) The effect of acute inflammatory episodes (cellulitis) on the treatment of lymphoedema. *J Tissue Viabil* **3**(2): 51–5

Jenns K (2000) Management strategies. In: Twycross R, Jenns K, Todd J, eds. *Lymphoedema*. Radcliffe Medical Press, Oxford: 97–117

Keeley V (2000) Clinical features of lymphoedema. In: Twycross R, Jenns K, Todd J, eds. *Lymphoedema*. Radcliffe Medical Press, Oxford: 44–67

Kirshbaum M (2000) Breast lymphoedema. In: Twycross R, Jenns K, Todds J, eds. *Lymphoedema*. Radcliffe Medical Press, Oxford: 321–30

Levick JR (1991) Circulation of fluid between plasma, interstitium and lymph. In: *Introduction to Cardiovascular Physiology*. Butterworth, London: 143–70

Ling J, Duncan A, Laverty D, Hardy J (1997) Lymphorrhoea in palliative care. *Eur J Palliat Care* **4**(2): 50–2

Mortimer PS (1990) Investigation and management of lymphoedema. *Vasc Med Rev* **1**: 1–20

Mortimer PS (1995a) Managing lymphoedema. *Clin Exp Dermatol* **20**: 98–106

Mortimer PS (1995b) The dermatologist's contribution to lymphoedema management. *Scope Phlebol Lymphol* **3**: 17–9

Mortimer PS (2001) Acute inflammatory episodes. In: Twycross R, Jenns K, Todd J, eds. *Lymphoedema*. Radcliffe Medical Press, Oxford: 130–9

Mortimer PS, Bates DO, Brassington HD, Stanton AWB, Strachan DP, Levick JR (1996) The prevalence of arm oedema following treatment of breast cancer. *Q J Med* **89**: 377–80

Pezner RD (1986) Arm lymphoedema in patients treated conservatively for breast cancer. *Int J Radiat Oncol Biol Phys* **12**: 2079–83

Price B (1992) Living with altered body image: the cancer experience. *Br J Nurs* **1**(13): 643–4

Shankar S, Marshall K, Mortimer PS (2000) Skin care in lymphoedema. British Lymphology Society Autumn newsletter, Sevenoaks, Kent **28**: 5–8

Stanton A (2000) How does tissue swelling occur? The physiology and pathophysiology of interstitial fluid formation. In: Twycross R, Jenns K, Todd J, eds. *Lymphoedema*. Radcliffe Medical Press, Oxford: 11–21

Tadych K (1987) Postmastectomy seromas and wound care. *Surg Gynecol Obstet* **165**: 483–7

Tortora G, Grabowski SR (1993) The cardiovascular system: blood vessels and haemodynamics. In: *Principles of Anatomy and Physiology*. 7th edn. Harper Collins, New York: 632–4

Veitch J (1993) Skin problems in lymphoedema. *Wound Manage* **4**: 242–5

Williams A (1997) Update: lymphoedema. *Profess Nurse* **12**(9): 645–8

Wilson C, Bilodeau ML (1989) Current management concepts for the patient with lymphoedema. *Cardiovasc Nurse* **4**(1): 79–88

Woods M, Tobin M, Mortimer PS (1995) The psychosocial morbidity of breast cancer patients with lymphoedema. *Cancer Nurs* **18**(6): 467–71

World Health Organization online at: http//: www.who.int/inf-fs/en/fact102.html

7

Evidence-based surgical wound care on surgical wound infection

Jacqueline Reilly

Surgical wound infection is an important outcome indicator in the postoperative period. A three-year prospective cohort epidemiological study of 2202 surgical patients from seven surgical wards, across two hospitals, was carried out using gold standard surveillance methodology. This involved following patients up as inpatients and post-discharge surveillance to thirty days by an independent observer. The results led to the development of a mathematical model for risk of clean, elective surgical wound infection. Risk of surgical wound infection was increased by smoking, higher body mass index, presence of malignancy, haematoma formation, increasing numbers of people in theatre, adherent dressing usage, and higher times to suture removal (P<0.05). The results show that this type of surveillance is an effective way of collecting accurate data on wound infection rates. It was noted that patient care practices affected the surgical wound infection rate and the surveillance was used to facilitate the adoption of evidence-based practice, through recommendations for clean surgery, to reduce the risk from extrinsic risk factors for wound infection. As a result of the implementation of this evidence-based practice there was a significant reduction (P<0.05) in the clean wound infection rate.

At any one time, around one in ten hospital patients has a hospital-acquired infection, with a minimum of 100000 hospital-acquired infections occurring each year (National Audit Office [NAO], 2000). This has serious implications for increased mortality and morbidity and the costs associated with treatment of these infections. Indeed, it has been estimated that hospital-acquired infection costs the NHS over one billion pounds per year, with an average increase in hospital costs of between £1618 and £2398 per patient with a surgical wound infection (Plowman *et al*, 1999).

Despite these negative effects of surgical wound infection, data about their incidence and risk factors are incomplete. A risk factor within the field of surgical site infection refers to a variable, which has a significant association with the development of a surgical wound infection postoperatively (Mangram *et al*, 1999). These factors include those which are intrinsic and extrinsic in the population. Intrinsic factors include: age; active skin condition; smoking status; body mass index (BMI); and comorbidity. Extrinsic factors, which are risk factors to the population include: pre-, peri- and postoperative patient care practices such as preoperative skin preparation; and postoperative dressings.

The focus of this chapter is on wound care specifically, thus the patient care practices associated with this will be discussed.

Surgical wound dressings

The evidence base for dressing choice is that wound dressings are employed to absorb wound secretions, protect the wound from injury, and protect the wound against bacterial contamination. Adherent dressings can increase the risk of mechanical damage to the wound when they are removed, thus leaving an entry site for bacterial contamination (Chrintz *et al*, 1989). Non-adherent dressings should be used on surgical wounds (Phillips, 2001).

The evidence base, with regard to removal of dressings, is that experimental studies have shown that a carefully sutured wound with haemostasis is sealed by fibrin within twenty-four hours. The wound thereafter becomes effectively protected against outside moisture and bacterial contamination (Heifetz *et al*, 1952; Lindsay and Birch, 1964). Wound dressings should therefore not be removed less than twenty-four hours after surgery because of the mechanical damage that can be done to the wound before this time (Chrintz *et al*, 1989).

Mechanical damage to wounds can lead to easy access for bacteria and, as such, could be an independent risk factor for surgical wound infection. Non-experimental, research-based evidence supports the removal of dressings on the second day postoperatively (Cruse and Foord, 1980), or a minimum of twenty-four hours postoperatively, and that wounds should be left exposed thereafter (Gilchrist, 1990).

Development of the study

Given the uncertainty, both at a national and local level, about the incidence of surgical wound infection, and the associated risk factors, it was decided to undertake an investigation: the aim of which was to identify if the risk factors identified in the literature were responsible for the clean wound infection rate. It was also proposed that by influencing healthcare professionals' postoperative wound care practices (extrinsic risk factors), the incidence of infection might be reduced.

Study population

The study population consisted of all general surgical patients undergoing elective clean surgery within two district general hospitals in one Scottish health board during a three-year period. Patients were identified from theatre lists. Data were collected from the two hospitals, encompassing five consultant surgeons and associated nursing staff based on seven wards.

Definitions

Surgical wound infection

The definition used for infection in this study was:

> *A wound infection should have either a purulent discharge in, or exuding from, the wound, or a painful spreading erythema indicative of cellulitis. Infection should be considered to be present when there is fever (≥38°C), tenderness, oedema and an extending margin of erythema, or the patient is still receiving active treatment for a wound which has discharged pus.*

> Emmerson *et al*, 1993

This definition was used in conjunction with a previously validated wound assessment scoring tool (Bailey *et al*, 1992) to enable a strict criterion to be applied, as scoring systems have been shown to be more objective and sensitive than using a definition on its own (Wilson *et al*, 1998).

Clean surgery

Cruse (1992) defined clean surgery as:

> *Clean wounds are those from operations in which the gastrointestinal, genitourinary, or respiratory tract is not entered, no apparent inflammation is encountered, and no break in aseptic technique occurs; however, three operations — cholecystectomy, appendicectomy in passing, and hysterectomy — are usually included in this category if no acute inflammation is present.*

> Cruse, 1992

The study concentrated on infections in 'clean' surgery (Cruse, 1992) because endogenous (patient's own normal flora at the site) bacterial contamination is at a minimum in these wounds and the influence of other risk factors affecting wound infection could thus be assessed.

Ethical approval

All data collection techniques employed were unobtrusive as they were obtained by recording of practice and from physical evidence requiring no alteration to the patient's usual treatment. However, ethical approval was sought and granted from the health board area ethics committee.

Inclusion/exclusion criteria

The study included all patients undergoing clean elective surgery involving a general anaesthetic. The study excluded patients undergoing minor clean procedures. Minor was defined as those operations involving local anaesthetic use only.

Method

Data were collected on both intrinsic and extrinsic risk factors. These risk factors are detailed in *Table 7.1*. A wound surveillance nurse, employed specifically for the surgical wound infection surveillance, collected data prospectively. Data on risk factors for wound infection for each patient were obtained using a data collection form including all the risk factors listed in *Table 7.1*. Data were collected from case notes and daily visits were made to the patient, while inpatient pre-, peri- and postoperative care was recorded and the wound was given a score using the wound infection assessment tool (Bailey *et al*, 1992). The wound surveillance nurse observed wounds after the ward staff had removed any dressings.

Table 7.1: Intrinsic and extrinsic risk factors included in the study

Intrinsic risk factors	Extrinsic risk factors
Age	Consultant
Sex	Ward
Postcode (social class/deprivation score)	Length of stay (preoperative and total)
American Society of Anesthesiologists	Preoperative shave type and time (ASA) score
	Preoperative wash
Risk assessment of specific comorbidity	Anticoagulant use
Smoker	Local anaesthetic infiltration to wounds
Body mass index	Prophylactic antibiotics
Active skin condition operation class	Theatre and number of people in theatre
Previous operation at same site	Previous dirty operation on list
	Prosthetic implant
	Surgeon and grade
	Duration of operation
	Drain type and drain removal date
	Dressing type and dressing removal date
	Closure type and suture removal date

Patients were reviewed postoperatively either at home or within special wound surveillance clinics set up within the treatment room of one of the surgical wards within each of the study hospitals. The final assessment of the wound was made thirty days postoperatively.

The baseline infection rate was determined within the first two months of data collection. Thereafter, the data on infection rates were collated, graphed, and reported anonymously to the surgeons and nurses participating in the study. The effect of this feedback on practice was noted and thereafter a planned change intervention, in the form of evidence-based guidelines for the prevention of surgical wound infection, was implemented. The effect of this intervention was also measured.

The intervention of evidence-based guidelines

The intervention within this study was guidelines for evidence-based surgical practice, which were introduced within a normative re-educative approach to change involving workshops for all healthcare staff involved. All surgical care practices were reviewed, many of which were already evidence-based in practice; however, a few required change in relation to wound care. The change to practice was thus to cease the use of adherent dressings, such as gauze swabs, to minimize mechanical damage to wounds, and to cease stripping of wounds on the first day postoperatively during the ward round, and instead remove dressings twenty-four hours postoperatively.

Results

Data were collected between 1 November 1995 and 31 March 1999. A total of 2241 clean elective surgical operations were included in the study; thirty-nine were excluded from the analysis because the outcome was indeterminable, leaving a sample of 2202.

The incidence of surgical wound infection during the study period was 10% (n=220). The initial baseline infection rate was 14% (22/157, representing the 157 operations that were performed during the 'start-up' period of the study); with the feedback of infection rate data to healthcare staff the rate was reduced to 10% (103/1000). This reduction was clinically significant, as fewer patients developed surgical wound infections. However, this reduction was not statistically significant. The reduction in the surgical wound infection rate from the baseline period (14%) to the period where practices were changed by introducing evidence-based guidelines for wound care (8%; 46/592) was statistically significant (P<0.05) (*Figure 7.1*).

A logistic regression analysis was performed on the data, using the model-building strategy described in Hosmer and Lemeshow (1989). Within epidemiology studies, regression methods are used to model the relationship between a response variable and one or more explanatory variables. The objective of this method is to find the best-fitting and most straightforward, yet biologically reasonable, model to describe the relationship between a dichotomous outcome variable (presence or absence of surgical wound infection) and a set of independent variables (risk factors).

Risk factors found to be at least moderately significant (P<0.25) at the univariate stage of the analysis are shown in *Table 7.2*.

Each predictor in this initial multivariate model was examined for statistical significance using the Wald statistic (Hosmer and Lemeshow, 1989). This resulted in successive removal from the model of several predictors, one at a time, until the model contained only significant predictors of surgical wound infection (ie. P<0.05). The resulting multivariate model contained the following variables: BMI; number of people present in theatre; time; stitches *in situ*; dressing type; haematoma formation; smoking; and comorbidity.

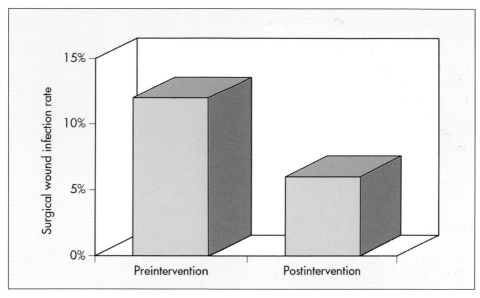

Figure 7.1: Surgical wound infection rates pre- and post-intervention of evidence-based practice

Next, all two-way interactions between variables were considered, as each was clinically plausible, eg. patients with a comorbidity of malignancy and having received chemotherapy. Only those interactions where the main effect variables were included in the model were considered (Nelder, 1998). This procedure found no significant interactions. As none of the two-way interactions were found to be significant, no further interactions were considered. The final fitted model was:

$$P(\text{wound infection}/x) = \frac{1}{1+\exp[-G(x)]}$$

Here, P(wound infection/x) denotes the estimated probability that a patient with characteristics 'x' will develop a wound infection (*Figure 7.2*). The 'x' characteristic may be smoking status, body mass index, diabetes status, etc.

As an illustration of the interpretation of the final equation, suppose we compare two patients who are alike intrinsically but have differing patient care practices carried out while in hospital: patient X has stitches *in situ* for more than ten days and an adherent dressing on his wound; patient Y has stitches removed between days five and ten postoperatively and a non-adherent dressing in place. Patient X's odds ratio of developing a surgical wound infection is 6.12 times that of patient Y.

Jacqueline Reilly

Discussion

The multivariate analysis has suggested that the variables which have an adverse influence on wound infection outcome are:

1. BMI
2. Presence of a haematoma
3. Adherent dressing usage
4. Smoking
5. Long skin closure times (>10 days)
6. Increasing number of people in theatre
7. Presence of malignancy
8. Use of chemotherapy, indicating increased likelihood of a surgical wound infection for patients with these characteristics relative to patients without them.

Table 7.2: Risk factors found to be at least moderately significant (P<0.25)

Length of stay (days)
Body mass index
Operation time (minutes)
Drain in place
Stitches in place (days)
Age (years)
Preoperative length of stay
Number of people present in theatre
Dressing in place (days)
Comorbidity
Anticoagulant
Operation class
Closure method
Dressing type
Haematoma
American Society of Anesthesiologists (ASA) score, drain in situ, surgeon consultant
Implant
Feedback of infection rate data to surgeons and nurses
Smoker
Prophylactic antibiotics
Sex
Preoperative shave
Another operation at same site
Preoperative wash
Grade of surgeon
Ward
Introduction of recommendations for evidence-based practice

Interestingly, the extrinsic risk factors found to be significant in the final model, namely dressing type and stitch removal day, were among the practice changes addressed by the evidence-based guidelines.

The risk factors found to be significant in the development of surgical wound infection within this study were comparable in part to some previously indicated in the literature. The risk factors of BMI and malignancy were found by some studies (Bibby *et al*, 1986; Garrow, 1988; Weigelt *et al*, 1992; Emmerson, 1998) to be important in terms of outcome. However, the risk factors of haematoma, smoking, number of people present in theatre, dressing type, and suture removal date are not commonly quoted in the literature. This may be due in part to their not being included in the dataset of other studies.

This study serves to illustrate how small changes to clinical practice in terms of postoperative wound care can have a big impact on outcome for the patient.

The model serves to describe the complex relationship of risk factors contributing to the development of surgical wound infection and the final equation allows interpretation of this risk in terms that make 'clinical sense'. This is a useful way of interpreting outcome measures, such as surgical wound infection, and could be of use for many other areas of practice in the same way.

G(x) = -6.0070 + 0.0690*BMI + 0.0791*(stitch day between 1 and 10 days)
+ 0.5158*(stitch day >10 days) - 0.1851*(comorbidity of one risk)
+ 0.8210*(comorbidity of malignancy) + 1.4408*(comorbidity of chemo-therapy)
+ 1.3751*(adherent dressing used) + 1.4951*(6–7 persons present in theatre)
+ 1.5551*(8–9 persons present in theatre) + 1.9047*(>9 persons present in theatre)
+ 1.2250*(haematoma present) + 0.4976*(smoker)

*=multiply by; each term in brackets takes the value 1 if true, 0 if false; BMI=body mass index

Figure 7.2: Final fitted mathematical model for the predicted probability of a patient developing a surgical wound infection

Conclusion

While generating new insight on surgical wound infection risk, this study highlighted at a local level many areas for improvement in clinical practice, which reduced the risk of surgical wound infection. The mathematical model demonstrates the influence of changing wound care practice in terms of using non-adherent dressings on surgical wounds and removing stitches before ten days postoperatively on the subsequent surgical wound infection risk.

The impact of evidence-based practice had a significant effect on outcome for patients in terms of fewer wound infections. The impact to the patient is financial in terms of paying for prescriptions for treatment of infection, and in relation to quality of life issues such as pain, anxiety, and suboptimal recovery resulting in slow return to work or social activities.

In order that we are clinically effective in our surgical care provision as nurses, we must ensure that our practice is evidence based. This is important to ensure that we provide the right care, for the right patient, in the right place and at the right time.

References

Bailey IS, Karren SE, Toyn K, Brough P, Ranaboldo C, Karren SJ (1992) Community surveillance of complications after hernia surgery. *Br Med J* **304**: 469–70

Bibby BA, Collins BJ, Ayliffe GAJ (1986) A mathematical model for assessing risk of postoperative wound infection. *J Hosp Infect* **8**(1): 167–72

Chrintz H, Vibits H, Cordtz TO, Harreby JS, Waaddegaard W, Larsen SO (1989) Need for surgical wound dressing. *Br J Surg* **76**(2): 204–5

Cruse PJE (1992) Classification of operations and audit of infection. In: Taylor EW, ed. *Infection in Surgical Practice*. Oxford Medical Press, Oxford: 1–7

Cruse PJE, Foord R (1980) The epidemiology of wound infection. A ten-year prospective study of 62939 wounds. *Surg Clin North Am* **60**(1): 27–40

Emmerson M (1998) A microbiologist's view of factors contributing to infection. *New Horizons* **6**(2): 3–11

Emmerson AM, Ayliffe GAJ, Casewell MW *et al* (1993) National prevalence survey of hospital-acquired infections: definitions. *J Hosp Infect* **24**: 69–76

Garrow JS (1988) *Obesity and Related Diseases*. Churchill Livingstone, Kent

Gilchrist B (1990) Washing and dressings after surgery. *Nurs Times* **86**(50): 71

Heifetz CJ, Lawrence MS, Richards FO (1952) Comparison of wound healing with and without dressings. *Arch Surg* **65**: 746–51

Hosmer DW, Lemeshow SL (1989) *Applied Logistic Regression*. John Wiley and Sons, Chichester

Lindsay WK, Birch JR (1964) Thin skin wound healing. *Can J Surg* **7**: 297–308

Mangram AJ, Horan TC, Pearson ML, Silver LC, Jarvis WR (1999) Guideline for the prevention of surgical site infection. *Am J Infect Cont* **27**(2): 98–135

National Audit Office (2000) *The Management and Control of Hospital-Acquired Infection in Acute NHS Hospitals in England*. The Stationery Office, London

Nelder JA (1998) How strong is the weak — heredity principle? *The American Statistician* **52**: 315–18

Phillips SJ (2001) Physiology of wound healing and surgical wound care. *ASAIO J* **46**(6): 2–5

Plowman R, Graves N, Griffin M *et al* (1999) *The Socio-economic Burden of Hospital Acquired Infection*. Public Health Laboratory Service, London

Weigelt JA, Dryer D, Haley RW (1992) The necessity and efficiency of wound surveillance after discharge. *Arch Surg* **127**(1): 77–82

Wilson APR, Helder N, Theminimulle SK, Scott GM (1998) Comparison of wound scoring methods for use in audit. *J Hosp Infect* **39**(2): 119–26

Key points

⌘ Surgical wound infection is a key outcome indicator of surgery.

⌘ Surgical wound dressings should be non-adherent.

⌘ Mathematical modelling serves to describe the complex relationships of risk factors and infection.

⌘ Sutures and other wound closure materials should be removed before ten days postoperatively.

⌘ Ensuring practice is evidence-based can reduce the risk of infection in surgery.

⌘ Surgical wound infection rates can be reduced using an active programme of surveillance.

8

Exploring methods of wound debridement

Mark O'Brien

Dead tissue, in the form of slough and necrosis, can if present in a wound, delay healing and promote infection. Debridement describes any method by which such materials are removed and, as a consequence, the potential to achieve wound healing enhanced. In this chapter, the author discusses the history of debridement, cell death, the nature of necrotic tissue and a variety of debridement techniques.

'Debridement' describes any method that facilitates the removal of dead tissue, cell debris or foreign bodies from a wound. Early descriptions of the process of debridement extend back to Hippocrates (c. 400BC), who advocated the use of compression bandaging to effect debridement of leg ulcers and recognized the detrimental effects of leaving devitalized tissue in wounds.

The word debridement itself derives from the French débrider, to unbridle, ie. to remove a constraint. The term was first used by Henri François Le Dran (1685–1770), who used 'an incision to promote drainage and relieve tension' for casualties of the battlefield (Helling and Daon, 1998). A more conservative approach to treatment of war injuries by John Hunter (1794), and the advent of antiseptics (Lister, 1867), led to the virtual abandonment of this practice. It was reintroduced during World War I by Antoine Depage, who extended the principles of incision and exploration to the excision of dead tissue (Helling and Daon, 1998).

Contemporary debridement of chronic wounds utilises a wide range of techniques and materials to assist the removal of dead tissue in order to promote healing and restore the bacterial balance (Sibbald *et al*, 2000). Before examining these techniques, it is necessary to understand why tissue death (necrosis) occurs and why debridement is necessary.

Cell death and chronic wounds

Chronic wound formation is primarily related to ischaemic events, ie. a reduction or cessation of the supply of oxygenated blood to tissues. These events include:

- capillary occlusion in pressure sores and the neuropathic foot
- arterial obstruction in the ischaemic limb
- a combination of fibrin cuff formation (leaked fibrin deposited on the outer capillary wall in the presence of high venous pressures), white cell trapping and oedema, limiting oxygen diffusion in venous leg ulcers.

Human cells rely on a consistent supply of oxygen to maintain function. In the absence of oxygen, energy production within the cell shifts to anaerobic respiration, triggering a sequence of events that leads ultimately to dissolution of the cell nucleus and cell death (Huether and McCance, 2000).

Appearance of necrotic tissue

The physical presentation of necrotic tissue is dependent on moisture content. Dry necrotic tissue (eschar) is black and leathery in appearance and if totally desiccated is rigid and hard (*Figure 8.1*). If moisture content increases, the eschar softens and moves through shades of brown, yellow and grey (*Figure 8.2*). In the constant presence of moisture, eschar will break down, form slough and ultimately dissolve as the body's own enzymes act on the dead tissue to effect removal. This process is known as autolysis.

Slough is yellow or grey, wet, stringy tissue that adheres to the wound bed and resembles the appearance and texture of mozzarella cheese on a pizza (*Figure 8.3*). Slough should not be confused with the yellow gelatinous coating of fibrin occasionally seen on superficial lesions (resembling melted cheese on toast) (*Figure 8.4*). This fibrin coating is not thought to impede healing and attempts at removal may lead to trauma of healing tissue.

There have been no randomized controlled trials (RCTs) examining the effect on healing of debridement *vs* no debridement of chronic wounds. Clinical experience, however, would appear to support the assertion that wounds containing necrotic material do not heal successfully and the National Institute for Clinical Excellence (NICE, 2001) has recognized that:

> *Debridement is an accepted principle of good wound care, especially when debris is acting as a focus for infection.*

It has also been suggested that the presence of necrotic tissue can 'splint' the wound (Baharestani, 1999), preventing closure by inhibiting wound contraction. In addition, the presence of necrotic tissue can generate malodour by supporting the growth of anaerobic bacteria, and obscure the wound bed making assessment difficult. Its appearance can be distressing to patients.

Methods of debridement

The main methods of debridement, which are discussed in more detail below, are:

- autolytic
- chemical
- enzymatic
- mechanical
- sharp.

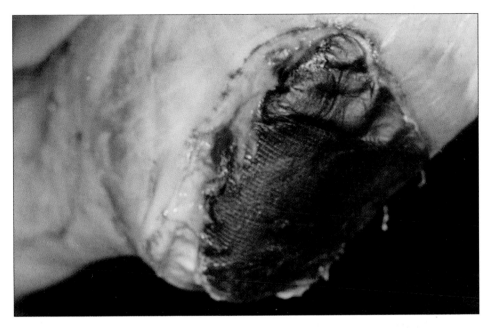

Figure 8.1: Dry necrotic eschar on a heel pressure ulcer

Autolytic

As already discussed, necrotic tissue will, if kept moist, gradually dissolve. The enzymes that facilitate this process are known as the matrix metalloproteinases (MMPs). MMPs are expressed by injured tissue and, once mobilized in the presence of moisture, are able to break down all elements of the necrotic tissue (Parks, 1999). The main dressing products used to promote autolysis are:

* films
* hydrocolloids
* hydrogels.

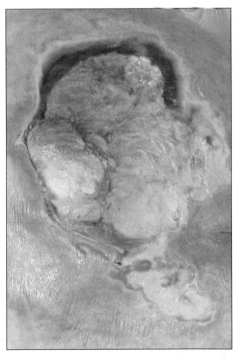

Films and hydrocolloids retain the body's own moisture while hydrogels donate water into the necrotic tissue. Due to the need for moisture to collect under films and hydrocolloids, in the author's experience they are generally slower at achieving debridement than the hydrogels.

Figure 8.2: Moist necrotic tissue

Hydrogels are typically composed of starch (natural or manufactured), water and a preservative. Differences in composition lead to variation in their fluid donating and fluid absorbing properties, altering their ability to promote autolysis (Thomas, 1994). A gel capable of donating large quantities of water into a wound may be ideal to promote autolysis but its reduced ability to absorb exudate can lead to maceration of surrounding tissues and poor dressing retention. Therefore, most manufacturers aim to achieve a balance between fluid absorption and fluid donation.

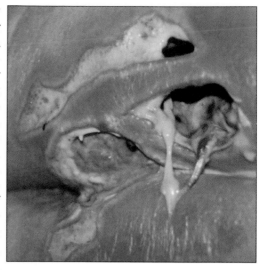

Figure 8.3: Slough

Autolytic debridement should be avoided when dealing with the ischaemic limb where the rehydration of eschar can activate bacterial spores, causing extension of gangrene and threatening the limb (Hampton, 1997). The objective in such circumstances is to desiccate the eschar using either dry dressings or povidone-iodine until revascularization of the limb is possible or mummification (stable but attached dry necrosis) or auto-amputation (separation of dry necrosis without physical intervention) of the affected area occurs.

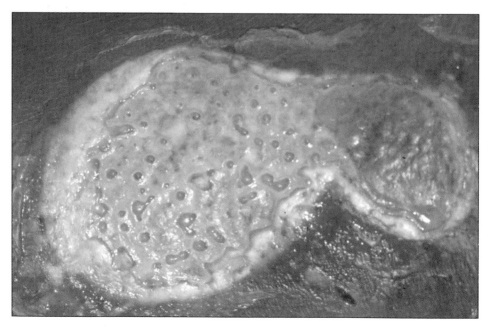

Figure 8.4: Fibrin coating on a superficial burn

Chemical

Historically a number of chemical agents have been used to promote debridement. The main disadvantages of most chemical agents are concurrent deleterious effects on healing tissue and irritant effects on surrounding skin. Therefore, the use of chemical agents in clean, non-infected wounds is contraindicated.

Malic/benzoic/salicylic acid combinations

Low pH leads to separation of dead tissue but may also cause maceration and irritation of surrounding skin (Morgan, 1997). There is no evidence that usage is more effective than gentler autolytic methods.

Hypochlorites (Edinburgh University Solution of Lime (EUSOL), Dakin's Solution, Milton®)

The hypochlorites are bactericidal but have been shown in animal studies to be toxic to healthy cells (Brennan and Leaper, 1987) and in practice to be caustic to healthy tissue and intact skin (Morgan, 1997). While their use persists in some clinical areas, hypochlorites have largely been superceded by less toxic agents.

Hydrogen peroxide (solution/cream)

Hydrogen peroxide solution has an instantaneous bactericidal effect, as it releases oxygen on contact with body tissues. A secondary reaction with the enzyme catalase produces frothing, which can flush debris out of the wound but has no effect on attached slough or eschar. Unfortunately, the concentrations required to achieve bacterial clearance (3%) are also toxic to fibroblast cells which are essential to wound healing. There is also a theoretical risk of air embolism formation (Morgan, 1997). The lower concentrations achieved by hydrogen peroxide cream (1.5%) provide a less toxic agent and its sustained release makes it a potentially more effective bactericide without damaging healthy cells.

Iodine

Povidone iodine (polyvinylpyrolidone iodine) is a water-soluble complex of elemental iodine and a synthetic polymer (Mayer and Tsapogas, 1993). Povidone iodine is an effective antiseptic, having a broad spectrum of activity against Gram-positive and Gram-negative bacteria, bacterial spores, protozoa, yeasts, fungi and viruses (Lawrence, 1998).

   Povidone iodine is available in solution (aqueous or alcoholic), ointment, spray and proprietary dressing formats. The alcoholic solution should only be used on intact skin as it will cause significant pain if applied to open wounds. The aqueous form is most commonly available in a 10% solution and is generally introduced into wounds in the form of a gauze soak. There is no clear evidence as to what the optimum concentration of iodine should be and in practice the concentration, duration and frequency of application tends to rely on the experience or whim of the clinician. Curiously, one *in vitro* study from 1982 demonstrated increased antibacterial activity associated with greater dilution (Berkelman *et al*, 1985). This suggests that in order to minimize the alleged deleterious side-effects of povidone iodine, lower concentrations could be used to greater antibacterial effect. Similarly, it could be argued that increasing the concentration would prolong antibacterial activity, as contact with exudate and absorption through tissue will gradually dilute the solution, increasing its effectiveness.

It is important to recognize the clinical objective of any plan of treatment. In the presence of infective necrosis, the primary objective is not to achieve healing but to preserve tissue and effect debridement. In my own clinical practice, 10% aqueous povidone iodine solution is used in cases of gross infection with associated tissue destruction. The application of povidone iodine appears to limit loss of tissue but, significantly, it also has a drying effect on sloughy tissue which facilitates sharp debridement (unlike autolytic methods which produce a wet, slippery, gelatinous slough that can be difficult to manipulate with scalpel and forceps). In conjunction with systemic antibiotics, this combination of therapies appears to effect rapid debridement (*Figure 8.5*) without adverse effects on the formation of granulation tissue. Once the wound is clear of necrotic tissue more conventional dressings adhering to the principles of occlusion and moist wound healing are adopted.

Cadexomer iodine can be used to similar effect (*Figure 8.6*). Cadexomer iodine is a three-dimensional starch lattice containing 0.9% iodine. The iodine is slowly released as the dressing absorbs up to six times its own weight in exudate and organic matter (Lawrence, 1998). A consensus group has suggested that cadexomer iodine may have a number of beneficial effects, including stimulating the healing process (Gilchrist, 1997).

Enzymes

The only commercially available enzyme preparation available in the UK is Varidase™ Topical (Wyeth Pharmaceuticals, Maidenhead), a product containing two enzymes: streptokinase (which dissolves fibrin clots) and streptodornase (which liquefies pus cells). Neither agent is effective at breaking down the collagen which forms 75% of the dry weight of skin (Baharestani, 1999). Given that the product is applied as a solution (or mixed with a gel under occlusion), it is difficult to separate the enzymatic effects from those of autolysis. Indeed, a small study comparing Varidase in a hydrogel and the hydrogel alone (Martin *et al*, 1996) showed faster eschar removal with the pure hydrogel, although the sample was too small to demonstrate a statistically significant difference. There is also a theoretical possibility of antigenic reactions in patients who have received or subsequently receive streptokinase for thrombolysis following myocardial infarction (Vowden and Vowden, 1999).

Other enzymes used in wound management but not available in the UK include, among others, bacteria-derived collagenase and papain-urea. Both products are capable of effecting the removal of necrotic tissue, however the selective debridement demonstrated by collagenase appears to favour its use over papain-urea, which can potentially damage healthy tissue and cause pain and peri-wound irritation (Falanga, 2002).

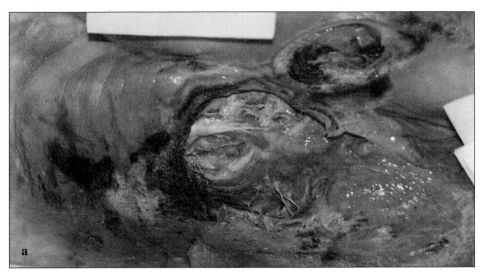

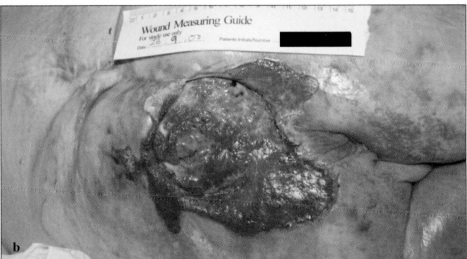

Figure 8.5: a) Grade IV sacral pressure ulcer on presentation; b) Grade IV sacral pressure ulcer after twenty days 10% povidone iodine soaks and regular scalpel debridement

Biological

Larval therapy (*Chapter 3*) describes a technique whereby sterile larvae of the fly species *Lucilia sericata* are introduced into a wound, where they secrete proteolytic ('protein-splitting') enzymes that break down slough and eschar, leaving healthy tissue intact. The resultant protein broth, together with any local bacteria, are then ingested resulting in a twenty-fold increase in larval size over forty-eight to seventy-two hours. The larval gut destroys the ingested bacteria, while other agents within larval secretions are believed to have an antibacterial effect on the wound bed (Thomas, 1997). Multiple case studies extolling the efficacy of larval therapy have been published (Thomas, 1996), but as yet no randomized controlled trials have been performed.

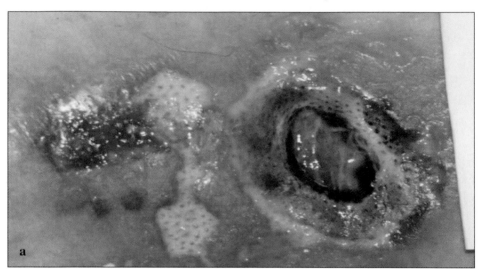

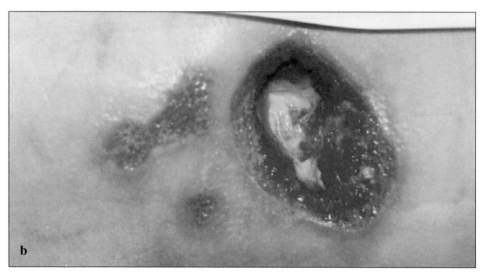

Figure 8.6: a) Grade III thigh pressure ulcer on presentation; b) the same pressure ulcer after twenty days 0.9% cadexomer iodine powder and regular scalpel debridement

Problems associated with larval therapy include:

- leakage of enzymes onto intact skin, which can cause temporary irritation and epidermal erosion
- the dressing procedure is straightforward once practiced but can be time-consuming
- unit costs are high in comparison to alternatives. However, the therapy can prove cost effective if rapid debridement is achieved.

Mechanical

Types of mechanical debridement include:

- wet-to-dry dressings
- high pressure irrigation or pulsed lavage
- whirlpool
- compression therapy.

Wet-to-dry dressings are now, thankfully, an historical footnote in British wound management but appear to remain common practice in the United States. The basic principle is to apply wet gauze to a necrotic or sloughy wound bed, wait for it to dry out and so adhere to the tissue. Once firmly stuck the gauze is pulled away along with the slough and usually a proportion of the underlying healthy tissue. As well as causing excruciating pain and reinjury to the patient, the gauze:

- does not provide a bacterial barrier
- may shed fibres into the wound
- does not provide thermal protection
- may disperse bacteria on removal.

In addition, despite low unit cost, gauze is not cost effective when compared to modern dressings (Ovington, 2002).

High pressure irrigation and pulsed lavage are rarely, if ever, used in the UK. They involve the use of high-pressure jets of water or saline being directed at the wound in order to loosen debris and remove bacteria. Specialist equipment is required to generate sufficient water pressure and protective clothing and a suitable environment required to cope with the subsequent splash-back of fluid, slough and bacteria.

Similarly, whirlpools are rarely used in the UK. In theory, the water softens the eschar and the turbulence helps to separate the dead tissue. In addition to the cost of the equipment and the logistics of immersing disabled patients, maintaining adequate infection control between patient immersions is a significant drawback of this technique.

Compression therapy

Compression therapy can act as an effective method of debridement for venous ulceration. Significantly, most pure venous ulcers do not present with an eschar but may develop slough in response to infective episodes or a prolonged inflammatory response. The action of compression in reversing venous hypertension, reducing oedema and providing a warm, moist interface for the wound generally leads to the separation of any slough without any secondary agent.

Conservative sharp debridement

It is necessary to differentiate between conservative sharp debridement and surgical debridement. Surgical debridement describes a procedure performed in an operating theatre under anaesthetic. All necrotic tissue is excised until only healthy tissue remains, or bleeding tissue is revealed, signifying adequate perfusion. Surgical debridement may also be applied to non-healing wounds where the surface tissue is excised to 'kick start' an acute phase of wound healing or prepare the area for skin grafting (Attinger *et al*, 2000). While in most circumstances surgical debridement is the ideal and definitive method of removing necrotic tissue, many patients may not agree to a surgical intervention or may be a poor anaesthetic risk by virtue of concurrent pathologies and therefore unable to undergo the procedure. There are also the added resource implications of theatre time and the availability of appropriate surgical staff to be considered, especially when dealing with patients in the community.

In contrast, conservative sharp debridement is performed at the bedside by appropriately trained and mentored nursing or medical staff. Tissue is removed in layers, using a scalpel or scissors, to just above the level of viable tissue. Rather than one definitive operation, the procedure may be staged in order to minimize patient discomfort and to allow deeper layers of necrotic tissue to demarcate following initial exposure. Conservative sharp debridement can be combined with other modalities (eg. autolysis, povidone iodine) in order to accelerate the process and remove remnants of debris not amenable to excision.

Conservative sharp debridement should not be a painful procedure, but patients may experience discomfort when slough/eschar is manipulated to allow excision and pulls on viable tissue. While no extra analgesia is usually required, some patients have innately painful wounds and will require additional pain relief. Adequate time should be given for this to take effect before starting the procedure. The use of topical anaesthetic (Emla™ cream, AstraZeneca, Luton) has been shown to facilitate pain relief during debridement (Rosenthal *et al*, 2001). However, Emla cream is not licensed for this purpose in the UK and it could be argued that if the patient experiences pain this indicates that viable tissue has been incised and provides them with protection from further damage.

Discussion

There is a presumption among clinicians that faster debridement leads to more rapid wound healing. While undoubtedly true in most circumstances, one does not necessarily follow the other. The injudicious use of chemical agents can have deleterious effects on healthy tissue (Brennan and Leaper, 1985) potentially impairing the healing process following debridement. However, restricting their use in all circumstances has its own pitfalls, particularly if translated to grossly infected lesions demonstrating active tissue destruction, where the primary objective is to prevent further tissue loss not to promote healing. Lack of consensus over the relative *in vivo* cytotoxicity of the various agents adds further to the confusion.

Although autolytic debridement is possibly the safest and easiest method of effecting debridement, it can be slow and has associated risks of maceration. Sharp debridement in contrast is fast and effective, but is an invasive procedure and carries a degree of risk. Anyone undertaking the procedure needs to:

- have undertaken training followed by a period of mentorship
- be aware of potential complications
- have a good understanding of local anatomy and underlying structures.

Two recent initiatives are aiming to support practitioners in these objectives. The *Nursing Procedure for Sharp Debridement of Wounds* (Fairbairn *et al*, 2002) is a guideline designed to provide nurses with a framework around which to base their practice of sharp debridement. The document is not cast in stone and users are positively encouraged to adapt it locally to the needs of their service. Tower Hamlets primary care trust conducts an annual three-day 'masterclass' in methods of wound debridement, which covers all aspects of debridement but has an emphasis on sharp debridement and includes surgical skills and cadaveric anatomy components. The course aims to provide nurses with the foundation knowledge and practical skills required to sharp debride. However, this groundwork must be consolidated through mentorship in their own clinical areas.

Careful selection of an appropriate method of debridement can prove pivotal in obtaining a successful outcome in the management of chronic wounds. Thorough patient assessment and an understanding of the materials and methods is essential if we are to remove necrotic tissue without delay or complication.

> **Key points**
>
> ⌘ Debridement describes any method that facilitates the removal of dead tissue, cell debris or foreign bodies from a wound.
>
> ⌘ It is generally accepted that the removal of dead tissue is essential if wound healing is to be achieved.
>
> ⌘ The principal methods used are autolytic, chemical, enzymatic, mechanical, sharp.
>
> ⌘ All methods of debridement carry an element of risk, it is therefore essential that the practitioner understands not just the methodology but also how it applies to the type of wound they are caring for.
>
> ⌘ Practitioners wishing to perform conservative sharp debridement should complete specific training and a period of mentorship before undertaking the procedure.

References

Attinger CE, Bulan E, Blume PA (2000) Surgical débridement: the key to successful wound healing and reconstruction. *Clin Podiatr Med Surg* **17**(4): 599–630

Baharestani M (1999) The clinical relevance of debridement. In: Baharestani M, Gottrup F, Holstein P, Vanscheidt W, eds. *The Clinical Relevance of Debridement*. Springer Verlag, Berlin: 1–16

Brennan S, Leaper D (1985) The effect of antiseptics and topical antimicrobials on the healing wound: a study using the rabbit ear chamber. *Br J Surg* **72**: 780–2

Berkelman RL, Holland BW, Anderson RL (1982) Increased bactericidal activity of dilute preparations of povidone-iodine solutions. *J Clin Microbiol* **15**: 635–9

Falanga V (2002) Wound bed preparation and the role of enzymes: a case for multiple actions of therapeutic agents. *Wounds* **14**(2): 47–57

Fairbairn K, Grier J, Hunter C, Preece J (2002) A sharp debridement procedure devised by specialist nurses. *J Wound Care* **11**(10): 371–5

Gilchrist B (1997) Should iodine be reconsidered in wound management. *J Wound Care* **6**(3): 148–150

Hampton S (1997) Wound assessment. *Prof Nurse* **12**(12): 57

Helling T, Daon E (1998) In Flanders' fields: The Great War, Antoine Depage, and the resurgence of débridement. *Ann Surg* **228**(2): 173–81

Hippocratic treatise on Fractures. Translated by Francis Adams online at: http://www.indiana.edu/~ancmed/fractures.htm [25th July 2002]

Huether S, McCance K (2000) *Understanding Pathophysiology*. 2nd edn. Mosby, Inc. St Louis

Hunter J (1794) *A Treatise on the Blood, Inflammation, and Gun Shot Wounds*. J Richardson for G Nicol, bookseller, London

Lawrence JC (1998) The use of iodine as an antiseptic. *J Wound Care* **7**(8): 421–5

Lister J (1867) On a new method of treating compound fractures, abscess, etc. with observations on the conditions of suppuration. *Lancet* **1**: 326–9, 387–9, 507–9

Martin SJ, Corrado OJ, Kay EA (1996) Enzymatic debridement for necrotic wounds. *J Wound Care* **5**(7): 310–11

Mayer DA, Tsapogas MJ (1993) Povidone Iodine and wound healing: A critical review. *Wounds* **5**(1): 14–23

Morgan D (1997) *Formulary of Wound Management Products.* 7th edn. Euromed Communications Ltd, Surrey

National Institute for Clinical Excellence (2001) *Guidance for the Use of Debriding Agents and Specialist Wound Care Clinics for Difficult to Heal Surgical Wounds.* The Stationery Office, London

Ovington L (2002) Hanging wet-to-dry dressings out to dry. *Advances in Skin and Woundcare* **15**(2): 79–84

Parks WC (1999) Matrix metalloproteinases in repair. *Wound Repair Regen* **7**(6): 423–32

Rosenthal D, Murphy F, Gottschalk R, Baxter M, Lycka B, Nevin K (2001) Using a topical anaesthetic cream to reduce pain during sharp debridement of leg ulcers. *J Wound Care* **10**(1): 503–5

Sibbald RG, Williamson D, Orsted HL *et al* (2000) Preparing the wound bed: debridement, bacterial balance, and moisture balance. *Ostomy Wound Management* **46**(11): 14–28

Thomas S (1994) Assessing the hydro-affinity of hydrogel dressings. *J Wound Care* **3**(2): 89–91

Thomas S (1996) Using larvae in modern wound management. *J Wound Care* **5**(2): 60–9

Thomas S (1997) The use of fly larvae in the treatment of wounds. *Nurs Standard* **12**(12): 54–9

Vowden KR, Vowden P (1999) Wound debridement. Part 1: non-sharp techniques. *J Wound Care* **8**(5): 237–40

9

To use or not to use? The debate on the use of antiseptics in wound care

Elizabeth Scanlon, Nikki Stubbs

The use of antiseptics for wound care has long been a controversial topic. This situation has arisen following reports of tissue toxicity upon exposure to high concentrations of some antiseptic agents in solution. Consequently, antiseptics gradually fell out of favour following the introduction of systemic antibiotics. Some antiseptics have a broad spectrum of activity that makes them effective against a wide range of microorganisms, including bacteria, fungi, yeasts and viruses. Recent renewed interest in antiseptics, as a result of the evolution of antibiotic - resistant bacteria, has led to the development of modern antiseptic dressings. This chapter aims to discuss some of these issues and set them in a practical context so that readers recognize the complexities of decision-making where the use of antiseptics is concerned. This, in turn, should enable a better-informed choice for practitioners.

The use of antiseptics in solution and dressing forms in wound care is controversial. Confusion among practitioners arises partly from the absence of clear and consistent guidance on their use. Where reliable research evidence is lacking, practitioners often rely on expert opinion for guidance — yet opposing arguments are frequently put forward by wound care experts and senior practitioners. Increased understanding of the arguments for and against antiseptics should help nurses in clinical decision-making. This chapter outlines some of the key considerations for planning the management of wounds using antiseptics.

Cape and Dobson (1984) define an antiseptic as 'an agent which tends to prevent the growth of organisms causing sepsis in wounds'. More recently, definitions have become increasingly detailed as expert knowledge around the effects of antiseptics at cellular level has increased. Antiseptics are now thought of as cleansing agents which affect cellular proteins. 'Antimicrobial' is the term used to describe the therapeutic use of agents such as antiseptics and antibiotics in preventing and treating infections (see *Table 9.1* for more detailed definitions).

History of antiseptics

The concept of 'putrefaction' or sepsis as a complication of traumatic injuries or surgical wounds has been known for hundreds of years. The term 'antiseptic' was first used by Pringle in 1750 in his study of the effectiveness of mineral acids in preventing putrefaction in wounds on dead animals.

Table 9.1: Definitions	
Term	**Definition**
Antimicrobial	Substances, including antibiotics, disinfectants and antiseptics, that are used to treat infections
Antibiotic	Substances capable of destroying or inhibiting pathogens and either derived from micro-organisms or synthetically manufactured
	Able to target selectively bacteria rather than viable tissue, so can be used in low concentrations
	Less toxic than antiseptics
Antiseptics	A disinfectant substance that can be used on skin and on wounds that either kills (cidal) or prevents the multiplication (static) of potentially pathogenic organisms. Antiseptics can be dilute disinfectants; they are not selective and therefore can be toxic to the host tissue — particularly at higher concentrations. Antiseptics have the advantage of rarely selecting for resistance, and being topically applied do not rely on the bloodstream for access to the wound. This is particularly important in ischaemic wounds.

Source: adapted from Flanagan, 1997; White *et al*, 2001

The antiseptic debate has been ongoing since Fleming's 1919 lecture to the Royal College of Surgeons about his work on antiseptics in septic wounds. He compared the use of iodine 2% with carbolic acid in field hospitals during World War I and found there were lower rates of gas gangrene in those treated with iodine.

Fleming described two types of antiseptics: 'physiological antiseptics' and 'chemical antiseptics' (Fleming, 1919). Physiological antiseptics were predominantly leucocytes and Fleming describes various ways of maximizing the body's own defences by altering the pH of the wound, removing slough and managing wound exudate. Increasing interest and knowledge in the physiological processes involved in healing is resulting in a resurgence of many of Fleming's ideas and is reflected in a number of so-called 'new' therapies, such as larval and VAC® (Vacuum Assisted Closure™) therapy.

Fleming also described some contemporary chemical antiseptics such as Edinburgh University Solution of Lime (EUSOL), Dakin's solution (sodium hypochlorite), carbolic acid, mercuric acid, iodine, flavine and brilliant-green. He considered three important aspects: a) their effect on bacteria; b) their effect on the leucocytes; and c) the duration of their effectiveness.

The use of antiseptics began to decrease when Fleming discovered penicillin in 1929. However, it was not until the early 1940s that fermentation processes enabled the large-scale production and use of antibiotics and for a time antibiotics became more popular than antiseptics.

Antiseptics continued to have a dominant role in the prevention and management of wound infection until the mid-1980s when the publication of seminal papers by Brennan and Leaper (1985) and Lineaweaver *et al* (1985) threw the nursing and, to some degree, the medical profession into turmoil. Brennan and Leaper looked at the effects of antiseptics on normal acute wound healing in rabbits and Lineaweaver *et al* used *in vitro* studies to look at their effects on fibroblasts. Both identified significant detrimental effects. However, these articles presented evidence on experiments conducted on clean wounds in rabbits' ears and generalized it to the use of antiseptics in all wounds on humans. Subsequently, antiseptics in solution became unpopular and were seen not only as unfashionable but by many as downright dangerous. They were excluded from clinical research projects for many years. More recently, following publicity on the development of antibiotic-resistant organisms, has focused attention on the value and use of antiseptics in both solution and dressing forms in the management of wound bioburden (Cutting, 2001).

How antiseptics work

Most antiseptics have a bactericidal effect due to a chemical reaction with proteins. However, as a result of their non-specific nature they will react with proteins in bacteria, human tissue, living and dead cells. Antiseptics are available in many forms, including soaps, solutions, ointments, creams, lotions and impregnated dressings. Their uses include skin disinfection, wound irrigation and cleansing, wound debridement and prevention and treatment of wound colonization and infection. *Table 9.2* summarizes the most common antiseptics. Due to their variety of uses and effects it is not surprising that nurses can become confused about when and why to use antiseptics. Dakin stated in 1915 that to:

> ... *make a judicious choice of antiseptic ... many different factors have to be considered in addition to germicidal activity, including the irritating properties of the substances, their toxicity, solubility, ability to penetrate tissues and to be absorbed, and their chemical reactions with proteins and other tissue constituents.*

Colonization and infection

To understand the appropriate use of antiseptics it is necessary to appreciate the differences between colonization and infection.

The presence of microorganisms in a wound is not unusual, but not all wounds support the same range and number of species (Cooper and Lawrence, 1996; Davies *et al*, 2002; Hill *et al*, 2003). Chronic wounds such as leg ulcers and pressure ulcers are usually colonized with a mixture of species, many of which can be potential pathogens. Kingsley (2001) proposed a wound infection continuum, where the wound can, under certain circumstances, progress from colonization to infection, and recommended certain actions to be taken at each stage (*Table 9.3*). One of the key recommendations made by Kingsley was to consider the use of antiseptic dressings at the critical colonization stage.

Application of Kingsley's continuum, together with an in-depth knowledge of the antiseptics available and their usage, should help to assist practitioners in their decision-making process.

The case for antiseptics

There is compelling evidence for the use of appropriate antiseptics in solution form for surgical site preparation, and in dressing form for the treatment of critical colonization and local infection. Some antiseptics are effective at destroying a wide spectrum of bacteria, fungi, protozoa and endospores (Cooper and Lawrence, 1996). In cases where the number of bacteria in a wound has increased to a point where it is detrimental to wound healing (ie. critical colonization), a product which is effective at reducing the bioburden and sustaining that reduction will be valuable.

Antiseptics are not given systemically; they are applied topically to the wound and the dosage is dependent on the type of preparation and the frequency of application by the professional, rather than relying on the patient complying with oral medication.

As antiseptics are applied topically, there are very few reported systemic side-effects. However, because of the limited amount of research regarding absorption of topical antiseptics it is unclear whether this absorption is detrimental. It is known that absorption increases with surface area treated, ie. when antiseptics are used on extensive wounds (Lansdown, 2002a).

From the evidence of epidemiological studies we know that some patients are more susceptible to infection than others (Cruse and Foord, 1980). Patients with diabetes, those with peripheral vascular disease or who are immuno-compromised for any reason are more likely to reach the point of critical colonization sooner and often proceed to a wound infection. Used prophylactically, antiseptics may potentially prevent infections for this type of patient and may prevent the need for systemic antibiotics. This is an important factor, given that compliance with antibiotics is poor and few patients take the full course (Kelly, 2001). This lack of compliance has also been linked to the development of antibiotic resistance. Some antiseptics are effective against antibiotic-resistant bacteria (*Table 9.2*).

Timely and appropriate use of antiseptics, based on an understanding of the pathophysiology of a wound and a skilled clinical assessment, may return a wound from critical colonization back to the state conducive to wound healing.

Bacteria in wounds can delay wound healing, and can also produce wound malodour. The toxins and other virulents factors, ie. invasins, produced by some bacteria may be destructive to the wound bed, causing an increase in slough and necrotic tissue. The presence of excess bacteria may cause an increase in the phagocytic action of the white blood cells and in the volume of serous fluid present in the wound. This leads to an increase in the amount of wound exudate. The use of antiseptics in this instance will have the additional benefits of odour management and reduction in exudate.

Table 9.2: Some commonly used antiseptics

Antiseptic	Indications for use	Spectrum	Adverse effects	Comments
Alcohols • Used either on their own (eg. isopropanol 70%) or for alcoholic solutions (eg. Betadine 10%)	• Skin and hand or hard surface disinfection	• All bacteria but not endospores	• Solutions fix skin cells and may cause irritation	• Should not be used on broken skin or open wounds
Chlorhexidine • 0.5% chlorhexidine tulle gauze dressing	• Prevention of colonization in superficial wounds	• All bacteria but not endospores, some viruses and fungi	• Occasional reports of severe allergic reactions	• *In vitro* evidence suggests poor release of chlorhexidine from the tule
• Solutions - (concentrations varying from 0.015%–5%, some combined with cetrimide, some requiring dilution	• Cleaning and disinfecting wounds	• As above		• Ensure appropriate solution is used
Dyes • Proflavine hemisulphate (0.1% solution or cream)	• Historically used with ribbon gauze to pack cavities	• Mildly effective against Gram-postive bacteria but less effective against Gram-negative	• Pain associated with dressing change and toxicity (DeMarini *et al*, 1988)	• No advantages over modern alternatives
• Potassium permanganate (1:8000–1:1000 solution)	• Used for astringent as well as antimicrobial properties to dry up macerated skin or excoriation due to varicose eczema		• Some reported allergic reactions, stains skin and clothing	• Little evidence to support use
Chlorinated solutions • Dakin's solution (boric acid, chlorinated lime and sodium carbonate giving 0.5% w/v available chlorine)	• Desloughing and sterilising of wounds	• All bacteria and viruses including endospores	• Delayed healing • Cell toxicity • Irritancy • Reduced capillary blood flow • Renal failure/ Schwartzman reaction • Hyperthermia and burns • Depressed collagen synthesis • Overgranulation • Localised oedema • Hypernatraemia	• Activity reduced in presence of - organic material and in alkaline
• EUSOL solution (chlorinated lime and boric acid solution containing not less than 0.25% w/v available chlorine)	• As above	• As above	• As above	• Only stable for two weeks once prepared
Hydrogen peroxide • (3% solution or Hioxyl cream containing 1.5% solution)	• Solution reacts with catalase causing frothing to help clean dirty, sloughy wounds • Hioxyl cream has prolonged antiseptic action (at least 8 hours)	• All bacteria especialy anaerobes	• Solution may be caustic to surrounding skin • Risk of oxygen embolus and surgical emphysema when used in body cavities	• May chemically interact with other topical medicaments • Contamination with organic material leads to loss of effectiveness

Table 9.2 continued: Some commonly used antiseptics

Antiseptic	Indications for use	Spectrum	Adverse effects	Comments
Iodine				
• Cadexomer iodine (0.9% w/w)	• Used for critically colonized or infected wounds or for desloughing	• All bacteria including endo spores plus fungal and protozoan cysts	• Not to be used on patients with iodine sensitivity or thyroid disease	• Bactericidal effect is reduced when in contact with organic matter • Iodine changes from brown to white/colour-less when deactivated
• Povidone iodine (iodine combined with polyvinylpirolodone which allows slow release of iodine)	• 10% solution used for skin cleansing • 10% impregnated viscose tulle dressing used for colonized superficial wounds • 2.5% dry powder spray used mainly for skin disinfection in dry ischaemic wounds	• As above	• Toxicity and delayed wound healing reported in clean granulating wounds	
Silver				
• Silver sulphadiazine	• Critically colonized and infected wounds, particularly burns	• All bacteria especialy Gram-negative, eg. *Pseudomonas* and fungi	• Allergic reactions to sulphonamides have been reported	• As the metallic silver is combined with an antibiotic, there is potential for developing resistance
• Silver impregnated dressings, eg. Actisorb Silver 220, Aquacel Silver	• Critically colonized and infected wounds; odour control and exudate absorption	• Effective against Gram-positive and Gram-negative	• None reported	• Some evidence from clinical trials.

Source: adapted from Pike (1983) and Cooper and Lawrence (1996)

Antiseptic dressings may be useful for disinfecting wounds before grafting; there is evidence that they are effective after grafting to enhance 'take' (Hansbrough *et al*, 1995). In plastic surgery, the ability of a graft to 'take' is dependent on the bacterial load of the wound. The risk of damage to any granulating tissue by an antiseptic such as EUSOL is outweighed by the benefits of the successful graft.

The administration of antiseptics in a slow or sustained-release form results in a prolonged antibacterial effect. Many modern antiseptic dressing products are sustained release (White and Cooper, 2003); this overcomes the problem of the antiseptic being deactivated in the presence of proteins (Lansdown, 2002b).

There is some research evidence to support the use of silver and iodine products for wound management (Mertz *et al*, 1999; O'Meara *et al*, 2000; Cutting, 2001). Systematic reviews looking for evidence of effectiveness of interventions in controlled trial situations have identified several studies which show evidence of effectiveness, but the trials are small and therefore not statistically significant.

Table 9.3: The infection continuum

Type of wound	Acute	Acute	Acute and chronic	Acute and chronic	Acute and chronic
Wound status	Sterile	Contamination	Colonisation	Critical colonisation	Infection
Wound bioburden	Absent	Usually low numbers with little active growth (high in some trauma wounds)	A relatively stable, dynamic equilibrium	Host defences unable to maintain colonisation	Increased levels of pathogens and invasion into host tissues
Microbial diversity (ie. variety of species)	Absent	Restricted, mostly transient species	Wide range of commensals and potential pathogens	Similar to colonisation	Restricted
Indicators of clinical infection	Absent	Absent, except inflammation associated with trauma	No overt host response	Some indicators present	Present
Antimicrobial intervention strategies	None	Wound cleansing and removal of devitalised tissue and inanimate objects from trauma wounds. Prevent further contamination in burns	Usually none, except reduce haemolytic streptococci and pseudonomads prior to grafting. Topical agents for odour control	Topical antimicrobial agents	Systemic anti-biotics +/- topical antimicrobial agents

Source: adapted from Kingsley, 2001

The case against antiseptics

While recognizing the value of antiseptics, practitioners must also understand their limitations. These are generally related to antiseptic solutions and their misuse.

Antiseptics are not selective between the cells of the pathogens and colonizing organisms, and the cells of human tissues. Concentrated solutions of antiseptics, such as EUSOL, are destructive to good healing tissue (Brennan and Leaper, 1985). Good knowledge and understanding of wound healing and management is required to restrict the antiseptic to damaged or non-viable tissue.

Antiseptics, whether in solution or in dressing form, are unlikely to be able to remove all bacteria when used topically. They will only be effective if not deactivated by proteins or neutralized by the components of exudate. Bacteria may also be present in tissues and on surrounding skin and will not be effectively eradicated by some antiseptics.

Due to their mode of action, the antiseptic properties of these substances are quickly exhausted. In the presence of protein-rich exudate or blood they may be virtually ineffective. Traditional antiseptic solutions, such as hydrogen peroxide and EUSOL are short-acting and are unable to maintain a microbicidal effect over time.

While traditional antiseptic solutions have a low unit cost, their cost-effectiveness has not been evaluated, as many require frequent dressing changes and involve high costs in terms of nursing time. In contrast, antiseptic dressings such as those containing silver or iodine have been shown to exert a prolonged antimicrobial effect, often up to seven days, indicating a likely cost benefit.

The variety of available antiseptic solution concentrations is likely to lead to inappropriate use. This is seen particularly with iodine solutions (Goldenheim, 1993), where different concentrations and solvents may lead to toxicity. Given that nurses are not chemists, this can be a concern to practitioners.

Where antiseptics are used to aid debridement, it may be difficult to isolate them to the unhealthy tissue. This argument is often used in the debate over EUSOL, whose damaging effects are well-documented (Brennan and Leaper, 1985). Although it is known to be effective in debridement, nurses have a responsibility to prevent unnecessary damage to the surrounding granulating tissue and skin. This can be protected with petroleum jelly or paraffin gauze.

Several side-effects have been attributed to antiseptics. Pain may be a problem and might be directly attributed to the chemical, as many studies (eg. Ormistron *et al*, 1985; Hansson *et al*, 1998) have identified links between iodine and pain. However, pain may be linked to the drying out of the antiseptic if it is dependent on a carrier medium for administration, eg. gauze and its subsequent painful removal. Systemic absorption may lead to problems, eg. hydrogen peroxide leading to air embolism, absorption of iodine affecting thyroid function and absorption of silver leading to skin staining (argyria).

Many prepared products have a short shelf-life and need to be replaced every two weeks.

Many experts warn about the risks of developing resistance to antiseptics and there have been some reports of this happening (Lansdown, 2002b). As yet, these are minimal compared to antibiotic resistance (Kelly, 2001).

Summary and conclusions

Antiseptics offer many benefits. Many of the initial problems with the simple preparations have been overcome with modern sustained-release dressing preparations. These provide effective broad spectrum agents such as silver and PVP-iodine, offering a sustained-release action which carries a reduced risk of side-effects. There is, however, an associated increase in cost of these preparations over the simple solutions.

Nevertheless, antiseptics are easy to apply as creams, ointments and dressings. They are often combined with familiar wound management products known to promote the optimum wound environment and enhance their benefits in colonized and critically colonized wounds.

These benefits of antiseptics are welcomed by many, particularly with increasing concerns over wounds colonized with antibiotic-resistant bacteria, such as methicillin-resistant *Staphylococcus aureus* (MRSA). However, to avoid excessive and inappropriate use, practitioners must ensure that they fully understand the modes of action of antiseptics as well as their indications and contraindications. These products are disinfectants and, if used inappropriately, many are toxic and dangerous. If used appropriately, they can be the key to wound bed preparation and promotion of healing.

Uncomplicated wounds are best managed using products appropriate to the presenting tissue in the wound bed — eg. sloughy or granulating — and maintaining the appropriate moisture balance. Where risk factors for infection are present or the wound is in a state of critical colonization, topical antiseptic dressings should be considered (*Table 9.3*). A nurse faced with a complex wound and considering the use of antiseptics should ensure that he/she has the appropriate knowledge of the risks and benefits of the range of products available.

However, given that our understanding of the indications for use of antiseptics in human wound management does not appear to have increased substantially since Alexander Fleming's days, it is clear that more clinical research is needed in order to direct our practice in relation to the use of antiseptics.

Key points

⌘ Antiseptic dressings offer a number of benefits for management of complex wounds; they have few risks and side-effects if used appropriately.

⌘ Due to the wide variety of antiseptic products and formulations available, their properties and the complexity of wound management, careful assessment is required to ensure appropriate treatment decisions.

⌘ A good knowledge and understanding of wound healing and management is required to ensure that antiseptics are used in a clinically and cost effective manner.

⌘ Further clinical research is needed to direct nursing practice in relation to the use of antiseptics.

References

Brennan SS, Leaper DJ (1985) The effect of antiseptics on the healing wound: a study using the rabbit ear chamber. *Br J Surg* **72**: 78–82

Cape BP, Dobson P (1974) *Baillière's Nurses' Dictionary* (18th edn). Baillière Tindall, London

Cooper R, Lawrence JC (1996) The role of antimicrobial agents in wound care. *J Wound Care* **5**(8): 374–80

Cruse PJE, Foord R (1980) The epidemiology of wound infection: a 10-year prospective study of 62,939 wounds. *Surg Clin North Am* **60**(1): 27–40

Cutting K (2001) A dedicated follower of fashion? Topical medications and wounds. *Br J Nurs* **10**(15): 9–16

Dakin HD (1915) On the use of certain antiseptic substances in the treatment of infected wounds. *Br Med J* **28**: 318–20

Davies CE, Wilson MJ, Hill KE *et al* (2002) Use of molecular techniques to study microbial diversity in the skin: chronic wounds re-evaluated. *J Wound Repair Regen* **9**(5): 332–40

DeMarini DM, Brock KH, Doerr CL *et al* (1988) Mutagenicity and clastogenicity of proflavin in L5178Y/TK cells. *J Mutat Res* **204**(2): 323–8

Flanagan M (1997) *Wound Management*. Churchill Livingstone, London

Fleming A (1919) The action of chemical and physiological antiseptics in a septic wound. *Br J Surg* **17**(25): 99–129

Goldenheim PD (1993) An appraisal of povidone-iodine and wound healing. *Postgrad Med J* **69**(suppl 3): S97–105

Hansbrough W, Dore C, Hansbrough JF (1995) Management of skin-grafted burn wounds with Xeroform and layers of dry coarse-mesh gauze dressing results in excellent graft take and minimal nursing time. *J Burn Care Rehabil* **16**(5): 531–4

Hansson C (1998) The effects of cadexomer iodine paste in the treatment of venous leg ulcers compared with hydrocolloid dressing and paraffin gauze dressing. Cadexomer Iodine Study Group. *Int J Dermatol* **37**(5): 390–6

Hill KE, Davies CE, Wilson MJ *et al* (2003) Molecular analysis of the microflora in chronic venous leg ulceration. *Br J Med Microbiol* **52**(Pt 4): 365–9

Kelly J (2001) Addressing the problem of increased antibiotic resistance. *Prof Nurse* **17**(1): 56–9

Kingsley A (2001) A proactive approach to wound infection. *Nurs Standard* **15**(30): 50–8

Lansdown ABG (2002a) Silver 2: toxicity in mammals and how its products aid wound repair. *J Wound Care* **11**(5): 173–7

Lansdown ABG (2002b) Silver 1: its antibacterial properties and mechanism of action. *J Wound Care* **11**(4): 125–30.

Lineaweaver W, Howard R, Soucy D *et al* (1985) Topical antimicrobial toxicity. *Arch Surg* **120**(3): 267–70

Mertz PM, Oliviera-Gandia MF, Davis S (1999) The evaluation of a cadexomer iodine wound dressing on methicillin resistant *Staphylococcus aureus* in acute wounds. *Dermatol Surg* **25**(2): 89–93

Morgan D (1993) Is there still a role for antiseptics? *J Tissue Viability* **3**(3): 80–3

O'Meara SO, Cullum N, Majid M, Sheldon T (2000) Systematic reviews of wound care management: (3) antimicrobial agents for wounds. *Health Technol Assess Rep* **4**(21): 1–237

Ormiston MC, Seymour MT, Venn GE, Cohen RI, Fox JA (1985) Controlled trial of Iodosorb in chronic venous leg ulcers. *Br Med J* (Clin Res Ed) **291**(6491): 308–10

Pike AW (1983) Antiseptic use in wound management. *Crit Care Nurse* Nov/Dec: 87– 93

White R, Cooper R, Kingsley A (2001) Wound colonization and infection: the role of topical antimicrobials. *Br J Nurs* **10**(9): 563–78

White RJ, Cooper R (2003) The use of topical antimicrobials in wound bioburden control. In: White RJ, ed. *The Silver Book*. Quay Books, MA Healthcare Limited, Salisbury

Skin changes in the at-risk foot and their treatment

Kate Springett, Richard J White

The skin provides a 'mirror' of the patient's general health, and any changes from normal for that person may be generalised or located to specific body sites. In the foot, poor quality skin may develop associated with a number of medical disorders such as diabetes or rheumatoid arthritis, and peripheral states such as peripheral vascular disease. In these instances, the foot is 'at risk' of developing ulcers following even minor trauma. To manage epidermal and dermal changes efficiently, it helps to have a good understanding of the skin structure and function as well as knowledge of the more common conditions affecting the poorly viable foot. Skin physical characteristics change in the 'at risk' foot and skin conditions and lesions, eg. anhydrosis, fissures, ulceration, can develop readily and, left untreated, there is increased morbidity and risk of mortality. Even apparently minor skin conditions in the foot are worthy of attention and appropriate treatment as introduced in this chapter, as all those involved in health care have a responsibility and role in foot health education.

The state of the skin reflects the general state of the body. The appearance of the skin and its appendages (hair, nails, sweat glands, sebaceous glands) and how it feels provide a clinical indication of well-being or ill-health of that person. Changes in the skin, nails and hair may be generalized or localized, eg. on the lower leg, foot or part of the foot. The foot that is 'at risk' of ulceration or other damage, and where there is the potential for slow or no healing can exhibit a number of features that are different from 'normal for that individual'. Early recognition of these features can mean prompt intervention and hopefully prevention of overt ulceration, to avoid the concurrent pain, distress and disruption of lifestyle.

Although methods of assessing the skin, nails and hair of the lower limb and foot are considered below, this assessment requires some expertise in interpretation. The information given is intended for the non-experienced clinician. If in doubt, it is wise to refer to the appropriate specialists.

Once any abnormal skin changes have been recognized, a decision needs to be made about whether these need some form of treatment. Understanding the mechanism by which a skin condition develops can help determine selection of the management plan and specific treatment, so an explanation of how the skin may develop various conditions is given. Again, it is wise to refer appropriately, but some 'first aid'-type methods of management are discussed, with clinical examples, which may form the basis of foot-care advice. Where there is evidence, the optimal method of management is given, otherwise the information noted is that which is in usual practice.

Skin anatomy and physiology

An understanding of skin structure and function is vital to the understanding of pathological processes and making decisions about what type of intervention is appropriate to the at-risk foot, and when this should be applied.

Hairy skin (*Figure 10.1*), which covers all the body except the palms of the hands and soles of the feet (*Figure 10.2*), is composed of an outer layer — the epidermis — and an inner layer — the dermis — with adipose tissue and fascia beneath (Marks, 1993). The dermis and epidermis are linked by the dermo-epidermal junction (or basement membrane). The epidermis has no direct blood supply, but has a few nerve endings, pressure-sensitive cells (Merkel cells), melanocytes (which govern skin pigmentation and offer protection from ultraviolet light), and Langerhans cells (involved in immunity). The dermis has a rich blood supply and a large number of nerve endings, particularly dense in the finger tips, to aid sensation and dexterity. Also within the dermis are hair follicles with attached sebaceous glands, and eccrine sweat glands (or apocrine sweat glands in the axillae). Hair in humans has a vestigial function in thermal insulation, and provides an indicator of health or disease. Sweat moistens the skin helping to maintain pliability, and also has a major function in thermoregulation. Sebum (secreted by sebaceous glands) forms a 'natural moisturizer' for the skin's surface.

Epidermal structure and function

The epidermis is a keratinized, stratified epithelial tissue and during the process of keratinization, the stratum corneum (the outmost layer of the epidermis) is formed. The stratum corneum is the body's primary barrier to the environment (Marks *et al*, 1985), minimizing opportunity for bacterial invasion (Misery, 1997), controlling incursion of toxins and allowing the body to maintain homeostasis (temperature, blood pressure control, etc.). During the process of normal keratinization, basal stem cells divide and the daughter keratinocytes move up into the rest of the epidermis (Wertz , 2000), and are eventually shed as small skin scales from the top of the stratum corneum (desquamation). The stratum corneum is not the inert, dead structure as once thought. It is capable of releasing some growth factors when traumatized (Brattsand and Egelrud, 1998) which will affect cell synthesis and cell turnover.

The skin on the plantar aspect (sole) of the foot and the palms of the hands (glabrous skin) has some structural and functional differences (*Figure 10.2*) compared with hairy skin. The stratum corneum in plantar skin is considerably thicker than that of hairy skin and has a different structure. It must withstand wear and tear (mechanical stress) more efficiently than hairy skin. Superficially visible are skin ridges — skin or finger prints. Eccrine sweat ducts open into the centre of the double ridges (Springett and Merriman, 1995). The combination of moisture from the sweat ducts and the skin ridging helps with grip (as car tyres do on roads).

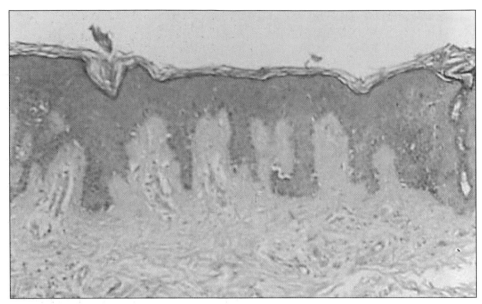

Figure 10.1: Light microscopic section of hairy skin (x40 stained with haematoxylin and eosis)

Normal plantar skin stratum corneum must be flexible and pliable to allow contact and conformability with contact surfaces. As no sebaceous glands are present in plantar skin, there is no natural moisturizing factor and plantar skin stratum corneum relies on the ability of its structure to retain optimal water levels (10–20% water; Potts, 1986) to maintain its flexibility. Sweating can be reduced in diabetes and peripheral vascular disease, changing the moisture content within the epidermis of the skin, so that it becomes less able to bend and cracks instead (fissures, *Figure 10.3*). The effects of exposure to sunlight and increasing age (Gnaidecka and Jemec, 1998) also change the skin's structure so that it has reduced conformability and restores less readily back to its normal position.

Dermis structure and function

Like the epidermis, the dermis too must be able to conform to contact surfaces, but also return to its normal state. It does this through its structure of fibrous proteins (collagen, elastin, reticulin) which are set within a matrix of a watery gel-like tissue (glycosaminoglycans). Collagen disorders like rheumatoid arthritis cause changes in the structure of collagen so that it is less able to take load. This means the skin on the plantar aspect of the foot is less 'strong' than usual and more easily damaged by the normal mechanical stresses of gait. Metabolic changes in diabetes affect the structure of collagen and epidermal keratins with resulting callus (hard skin) formation (Jude and Boulton, 1998; Hashmi, 2000). Presence of callus should be taken as herald or an advance warning sign of potential ulceration in diabetes mellitus (Edmonds and Foster, 2000).

If microangiopathy (small vessel disease) and macroangiopathy (large vessel disease) are present (eg. with diabetes or peripheral vascular disease), then the blood supply to the dermis is reduced. The nutrient and oxygen supply to the tissues fall, and metabolite removal is inefficient. The consequences are; that the tissues of the leg or foot can be painful (Humphreys, 1999), are at risk of developing ulceration, and have a reduced ability to handle infection (Frykberg, 1998). Lack of dermal blood supply also means reduced nutrient supply and metabolite removal for the epidermis.

The sensory nerve supply to the foot may be damaged in a number of disorders (eg. diabetes, Hansen's disease, sometimes in rheumatoid arthritis, multiple sclerosis, injury, etc.). If the protective sensation of pain is lost (sensory neuropathy), then the injurious effects of

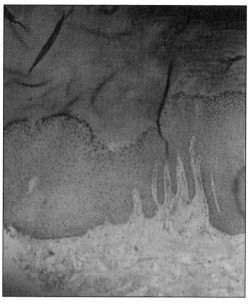

Figure 10.2: Light microscopic section of normal plantar skin (x40, stained with haematoxylin and eosin). The structure of the skin in this site can be seen to be very different from hairy skin

excessive heat, chemicals (eg. from keratolytic medicated corn plasters), or excess mechanical stress will not be perceived (Jude and Boulton, 1998; Edmonds and Foster, 2000). Excess mechanical stress, poor tissue viability, and neuropathy can lead easily to tissue damage (*Figures 10.3, 4, 5*).

Factors affecting tissue viability of the foot

Poor nutrition

Poor nutrition can make foot tissues susceptible to damage as poor quality skin structures are formed which are less robust than in healthy skin. Once the skin is damaged, nutritional status will also have an impact on healing. Poor nutrition can be the result of a wide range of factors which may be more prevalent in the older population, including:

- reduced social interaction
- immobility
- malabsorption syndromes (eg. following gastrectomy, pernicious anaemia)

- lack of awareness of nutrition requirements
- loss of interest in food.

Managing complex nutrition, and any associated psychological problems will require referral to an appropriate specialty, eg. nutritionist/dietitian.

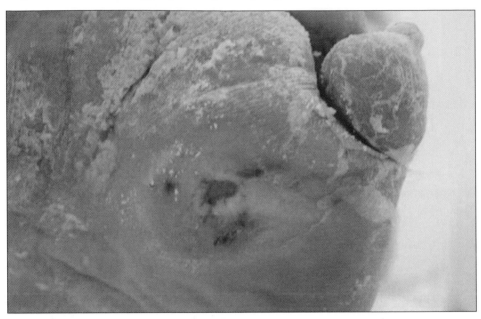

Figure 10.3: The plantar aspect of this foot shows anhydrosis (dryness), some dry fissures, and a neuropathic ulcer which tracks deep, distally and medially by about 2cm

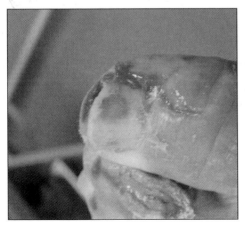

Figure 10.4: This neuropathic ulcer on the toe was caused by a hot water bottle burn

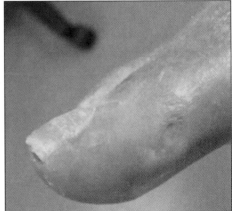

Figure 10.5: This foot is ischaemic and the small ulcer is extremely painful

Drug therapies

Some drug therapies can affect the quality of foot skin, making it fragile and more easily injured, for example, the corticosteroids. If skin changes are severe it may be appropriate to ask a patient's GP or specialist for an alternative therapy.

Medical disorders

Many medical disorders affect the skin of the foot, just as they would over the rest of the body. The skin, nails (*Figure 10.6*) and hair provide a mirror of what is happening to tissues that cannot be observed directly. Commonly seen changes in the foot related to medical disorders are given in *Table 10.1*. Differential diagnosis is often difficult, necessitating referral to the GP or specialist.

Dermatological conditions

Primary skin conditions such as eczema, psoriasis, contact dermatitis, viral, bacterial or fungal infections can affect the skin of the foot (Dawber *et al*, 2001) (*Figure 10.7*). All result in skin abnormality which may affect its barrier function and its mechanical integrity. Even minor damage in such conditions can result in a breach in the skin, with potential for infection and, in an at-risk person, delayed healing.

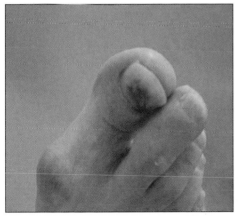

Figure 10.6: This nail has separated from the anil bed (onycholysis) which may have a history of trauma, be associated with thyroid disorders or dermatological conditions, such as psoriasis

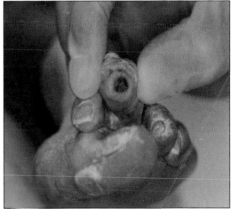

Figure 10.7: An interdigital corn has broken down into an ulcer with possible pseudomonal infection

In poor tissue viability, healing can be delayed by weeks, months and sometimes years, and often marked scarring results (Beldon, 1999). Scar tissue is weaker than normal tissue and there is an increased risk of re-ulceration at the same site. In the foot, this will need specialist care from a podiatrist and perhaps physiotherapist.

Footwear

Poor footwear (shoes, socks, tights, slippers) can precipitate callus and corn formation (hyperkeratosis) which often heralds tissue breakdown (Murray *et al*, 1996). Even when no hyperkeratosis is present, pressure from footwear can cause ischaemic changes predisposing to ulceration. These changes include blanching, hyperaemia, pain, anhydrotic scaling and reduction in the skin's normal resilient tone. Foot health promotion, including providing information on fit and style, is a key role for anyone involved in patient care, and a podiatrist can provide additional advice if required.

Foot function

Foot structure and function is strongly influential in ulcer formation, particularly in an at-risk foot. A foot which takes too great a load predominantly on one site, and for too long a duration, is likely to show ischaemic changes. This is a particular problem in a diabetic neuropathic foot when the warning sensation of pain is absent and tissue may be stiffer than normal owing to non-enzymatic glycosylation (Frykberg, 1998; Murray *et al*, 1996). The individual concerned is often unaware of developing foot problems. Ensuring footwear is suitable and has no rough or bumpy lining is essential, and foot biomechanics need to be managed by a podiatrist.

Assessing the at-risk foot and skin changes

Assessment needs to encompass the whole person, their general health, psychosocial issues, and their expectations of the assessment and treatment (Munro and Edwards, 1995; Merriman and Tollafield, 1995). Many skin conditions affecting the at-risk foot (*Table 10.1*) have similar features (Lucke *et al*, 2002; Dawber *et al*, 2001) and it is important to carry out a good assessment (Springett and Merriman, 1995) to help make a differential diagnosis and final diagnosis. This includes taking a good social and medical and drug history, along with analysis of clinical observations and tests:

- vascular system (large and small vessels, arterial, capillary, venous and lymphatics)
- nervous system (sensory, motor and autonomic)
- musculo-skeletal system
- skin (general and peripheral state, specific lesions and their spread)
- footwear and activity levels
- medical, surgical and social history.

Obtaining a good history is often key to the diagnosis, along with observation and tests (a useful mnemonic is HOT— history, observation, tests) (Merriman and Tollafield, 1995). It is worthwhile asking relevant questions, for example:

- how long have you had the skin/nail condition?
- have you had this before?
- if there are symptoms, what are these and when do they occur?
- are there signs of the same condition on other parts of your body?
- do you have any theories about the cause of the condition?

Observation of the general skin state, peripheral appearance and inspection of specific lesions is necessary. Comparison with contra-lateral or more proximal skin sites will help with assessment. Skin conditions can vary considerably and a diagnosis may not be clear, necessitating referral to the appropriate person or specialty.

Clinically accessible tests to aid diagnosis include:

- ankle brachial pressure index (ABPI) (Baker and Rayman, 1999) to assess arterial function
- doppler, to assess arterial (and venous) function
- checking sensation at different sites in the foot (10g monofilament, equivalent to Semmes Weinstein 5.07 filament), to assess peripheral neuropathy
- skin or nail scrapings to check for fungal infection
- swabs to check for infection.

Nail conditions (*Figures 10.5, 6, 8*) can also be seen in the at-risk foot, and these can be used to help with diagnosis of the condition (Samman, 1995; Springett and Merriman, 1995), although they may also be the result of unrelated conditions. Thin, brittle (atrophic) nails may be associated with poor peripheral blood supply, or clubbed nails with cyanotic heart disease. Thickened, ridged nails (onychauxis) often develop following trauma, either repeated minor, or major such as stubbing the toe badly. Spoon-shaped nails (koilonychia) can be seen in iron deficiency anaemia. Splinter haemorrhages in nails may be trauma-related or associated with rheumatoid arthritis or sub-acute bacterial endocarditis.

Managing the at-risk foot

Having assessed, considered differential diagnoses and possibly formed a diagnosis, clinical decisions need to be made in the light of national and local guidelines, and evidence- and knowledge-based practice. Management should include a patient-centred approach (Department of Health, 2000) as well as practical application of theoretical and experiential knowledge (Ryan, 1998). It is wise to refer the patient to the appropriate specialist, via their GP as appropriate, rather than waste the individual's time and effort, and cost to the NHS by inappropriate and prolonged 'dabbling'. Given the choice of an accessible specialist managing their medical or foot problem rather than a local generalist, it is probable that many people would choose the former.

However, difficulty comes in identifying when some people and their foot problems should be referred, and to whom. There are few foot health measurement tools or health gain indicators which are relevant to the general population (Gripton, 2002); many being specific to the diabetic (Hutchinson *et al*, 2000) or rheumatoid foot. Other difficulties that arise include barriers to communication, variation in NHS service provision across the country, increase in lay referral, and occasionally a tendency for practitioners to continue to care for an individual rather than accepting possible threat in referring the patient to another. The practitioner will need to make themselves familiar with local guidelines, routes of referral and specialist services locally.

A generally held 'rule of thumb' relating to referral time is that if a condition in an at-risk person shows little or no sign of resolution within, say, ten to fourteen days, then they should be referred to their GP, state registered chiropodist/podiatrist, specialist nurse (eg. tissue viability, diabetes), or medical specialist (eg. rheumatology, vascular, diabetes). Suspected or overt infection of the foot requires urgent same-day attention. *Table 10.1 (pp.130-131)* notes some management approaches for foot conditions which can predispose to further problems, including ulceration and infection. In addition, health promotion, foot health education and self-help are of great value.

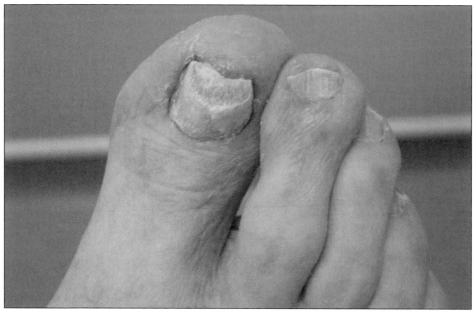

Figure 10.8: The differential diagnosis for this nail condition includes onychomycosis (fungal infection), onychauxis (thickening of the nail due to minor repetitive trauma), Darier's disease, sarcoidosis

What advice can be given to people whose feet are 'at risk'?

Every person has their individual needs and expectations of treatment, but nevertheless information on how to help ourselves is usually valued, for many different reasons including empowerment, reduced cost or time. Many of the specialist organizations (eg. Society of Chiropodists and Podiatrists, Diabetes UK, Tissue Viability Society) have footcare leaflets containing greater detail than that provided here. However, *Box 10.1* gives some general advice that the practitioner can give to the person with at-risk feet.

- Seek help and advice early: It is advisable to seek help from an appropriately qualified person such as a state registered chiropodist/podiatrist (SRCh, DPodM, MChS), clinical nurse specialist in tissue viability or diabetes, pharmacist or GP
- Check legs and feet frequently (ideally daily or more often): If a skin or nail problem is found following checking feet on a daily basis, the person concerned can be advised to apply a dry dressing (gauze, low adherent dressing) to keep it protected from further mechanical stress and to minimize the chance of infection. Hydrocolloid wafers (eg. ulcer dressings, blister patches or callus patches) can be helpful but only if instructions are followed closely (Springett *et al*, 1997) and there is contention in the use of hydrocolloid dressings in neuropathic feet (Lithner, 1990). With poor sensation, especially if the dressing is left *in situ* for too long, unperceived tissue breakdown can develop. If the skin is very fragile, then whatever dressing is used may need to be bandaged in place rather than being stuck in position with adhesive tape. The sufferer should be advised to seek help promptly
- Good hygiene: Keep feet clean and make sure the skin between toes is dry before putting socks, tights or stockings on
- Shoes, slippers and socks should fit well: Make sure footwear fits. Footwear should not be too small (or too large), too narrow or too shallow across the toe or foot. An easy way to check is to draw around the foot and match this against the size and shape of the shoe. If your shoes, slippers or socks have any bumps or rough seams, do not wear them
- Avoid extremes of temperature: Try to avoid extremes of temperature. If it is cold outside, let feet warm up gradually, don't use a hot water bottle or put them on a radiator. Check water temperature before jumping into a bath
- Topical applications: If the skin is dry, it can be helpful to apply an emollient (a cream to hydrate the skin), but be careful about keeping the skin between the toes dry, so this area does not become white and soggy (macerated)
- Avoid using 'medicated' corn and callus dressings, as potential for damage (eg. ulceration) to skin increases in the at-risk foot

Box 10.1: Advice to patients with an at-risk foot

Conclusion

A foot which has poor tissue viability is at risk of developing infection and ulceration causing pain and distress, and cost to the individual and society. A number of factors may be influential in the development of this state including medical disorder, poor nutrition and self-harm (eg. insistence on wearing footwear that does not fit). There is a wide range of conditions that can complicate the at-risk foot, and often differential diagnosis is difficult necessitating referral, via the GP, to the appropriate specialist. Nevertheless, all those involved in caring for someone who has at-risk feet have an essential role to play in provision of foot health education. Helping to prevent development of foot problems, to minimize complications with those conditions that do form and referring promptly before the condition becomes chronic is key to managing the at-risk foot. This requires assessment skill, experience and a sense of self-worth to relinquish care of a patient to another who has appropriate specialist knowledge and skills.

Key points

⌘ Factors influencing development of the at-risk foot include medical disorder, nutrition, peripheral blood and nerve supply, foot structure and function, footwear.

⌘ Complications of the at-risk foot are infection, ulceration, pain, distress, loss of social interaction, immobility, cost.

⌘ Patient should be referred on to the appropriate specialist rather than delaying.

⌘ All involved in care of the at-risk foot have a role in foot health education.

⌘ Specialists who may be involved in managing the at-risk foot include state registered chiropodists/podiatrists, nutritionists/dietitians, nurse specialists (eg. DNS, TVNS), medical specialties (eg. vascular, diabetes, rheumatology).

⌘ All health professionals should be familiar with relevant national and local guidelines and routes of referral.

References

Baker N, Rayman G (1999) Clinical evaluation of Doppler signals. *Practical Diabetes* **2**(1): 22–3

Beldon P (1999) Management of scarring. *J Wound Care* **8**(10): 509–12

Brattsand M, Egelrud T (1998) Purification and characterization of interleukin 1 beta from human plantar stratum corneum. *Cytokine* **10**(7): 506–13

Dawber R, Bristow I, Turner W (2001) *Text Atlas of Podiatric Dermatology.* Martin Dunitz, London

Department of Health (2000) *The NHS Plan: A Plan for Investment, A Plan for Reform.* The Stationery Office, London

Edmonds M, Foster A (2000) *Managing the Diabetic Foot.* Blackwell Science, London

Frykberg RG (1998) Diabetic foot ulcers: current concepts. *J Foot Ankle Surg* **37**: 441–6

Gnaidecka M, Jemec G (1998) Chronologic and photoageing due to accumulating effects of UVR. *Br J Dermatol* **139**(5): 815–21

Gripton J (2002) *Development and validation of the foot health and activities questionnaire: a podiatric outcome measure.* PhD thesis, University of Brighton

Hashmi F (2000) Non-enzymatic glycation and the development of plantar callus. *Br J Podiatry* **3**(4): 91–4

Humphreys W (1999) The red, painful foot: inflammation or ischaemia? *Br Med J* **318**(7188): 925–6

Hutchinson A, McIntosh A, Feder G, Home PD, Young R (2000) *Clinical Guidelines for Type 2 Diabetes: Prevention and Management of Foot Problems.* Royal College of General Practitioners, London

Jude E, Boulton A (1998) Foot problems in diabetes mellitus. *Br J Podiatry* **1**(4): 117–20

Lithner F (1990) Adverse effects on diabetic foot ulcers of highly adhesive hydrocolloid adhesive dressings. *Diabetes Care* **13**(7): 814–5

Lucke T, Munro C, Roberts D, Springett K (2002) Dermatological conditions of the foot and leg. In: Lorimer D, French G, O'Donnell M, Burrow JG, eds. *Neale's Disorders of the Foot.* Churchill Livingstone, Edinburgh: 197–257

Marks R (1993) *Roxborough's Common Skin Diseases.* Chapman and Hall Medical, London

Marks R, Barton C, Edwards C (1985) *The Physical Nature of Skin.* MTP Press, Lancaster

Merriman L, Tollafield D (1995) *Assessment of the Lower Limb.* Churchill Livingstone, Edinburgh

Misery L (1997) Skin immunity and the nervous system. *Br J Dermatol* **137**(6): 843–50

Munro J, Edwards C (1995) *Macleod's Clinical Examination.* 9th edn. Churchill Livingstone, Edinburgh,

Murray HJ, Young MJ, Hollis, S, Boulton AJM (1996) Association between callus formation, high pressure and neuropathy in diabetic foot ulceration. *Diabet Med* **13**: 979–82

Potts R (1986) Stratum corneum hydration: experimental techniques and interpretation of results. *J Soc Cosmet Chem* **37**: 9–37

Ryan T (1998) Evidence-based medicine: a critique. *J Tissue Viability* **8**(2): 7–8

Samman PD, Fenton DA (1995) *The Nails in Disease.* William Heinemann, London

Springett K, Merriman L (1995) Assessment of the skin and its appendages. In: Merriman L, Tollafield D, eds. *Assessment of the Lower Limb.* Churchill Livingstone, Edinburgh: 191–225

Springett K, Deane M, Dancaster P (1997) Treatment of corns, callus and heel fissures with a hydrocolloid dressing. *Br J Podiatric Med* **52**(7): 102–4

Wertz PW (2000) Lipids and barrier function of the skin. *J Acta Derm Venereol Suppl* **208**: 7–11

Table 10.1: Skin changes which may be seen in an at-risk foot with some differential diagnoses, clinical significance and indication of management/referral route

Skin changes in an at-risk foot	Examples of associated medical disorder or abnormality. Generalized peripheral state (area >5cm)	Associated with abnormality or medical disorder. Discrete lesions, or affected area (area <5cm)	Clinical significance and possible clinical management
Colour			
Erythema (red)	Infection, acute trauma, ischaemia (eg. associated with diabetes), bleeding, early bruising, gout	Vasculitis (eg. associated with rheumatoid arthritis), infection, hyperaemia following prolonged compression, extravasation, (blood forced into the epidermis), bursitis, a number of dermatological conditions (eg. pyogenic granuloma, psoriasis)	May need to observe over a day or two or ask patient/carer to observe, or refer to GP, state registered chiropodist/podiatrist (SRCh), specialist nurse, promptly or with less urgency depending on severity, history and provisional diagnosis. Dress lesion as appropriate (ie. low adherent gauze, antiseptic if relevant, bandage in place rather than adherent gauze, anti-antiseptic if relevant, bandage in place rather than tape if skin is fragile
Cyanosis (blue)	Venous impairment, heart disease, hypothermia, shoe dye	Chilling, chilblains, bruising, varicose veins	Treat chilling, chilblains with insulating insoles (if enough room in foot-wear), maintain constant temperature, avoid drafts. Anti-chilblain creams may help. Foam/cushioning pad or insole for bruising, if space in footwear. Refer to state registered chiropodist/podiatrist if no improvement in foot condition after a few days
White (blanching)	Acute arterial occlusion, Raynaud's phenomenon	Atrophe blanche, scarring, blanching from pressure, maceration, gouty tophi, application of medicated corn plaster (causes a chemical maceration associated with tissue breakdown	Foot health education (any practitioner) — is all footwear long, wide and deep enough? Protect, eg. scarring, maceration, pressure area if site looks fragile with dressing. Long-term care probably needed, refer to SRCh, TVNS or specialist department
Yellow	Slough (infected or aseptic), jaundice	Slough (infected or aseptic), callus, corn, exudate, xanthoma, gouty tophi, scarring	Routine cleansing of site, dress as appropriate, refer to SRCh for treatment or TVNS, DNS, GP for antibiotics if necessary.
Black/brown/grey	Shoe dye	Necrosis, scab from exudate, shoe dye, sub-epidermal maceration associated with tissue breakdown	If ischaemic, do not wet. Dry dress, refer promptly to SRCh for treatment or TVNS, DNS, GP for antibiotics if necessary
Green	Shoe dye	Pseudomonas infection	Dress as appropriate, refer to SRCh for treatment or TVNS, DNS, GP for antibiotics as necessary
Temperature Normally a gentle gradient of warm to cool, proximal to distal	Bilateral marked temperature differences — consider surrounding temperature and hypothermia, clinical shock ischaemic changes (macro- and microangiopathy), poor insulation by footwear, chilling, Raynaud's phenomenon	Patches of raised temperature — consider infection, friction/shear stress, RA flare-up Charcot's foot, thrombosis, chilblains	As for colour — erythema

continued

Table 10.1 continued: Skin changes which may be seen in an at-risk foot with some differential diagnoses, clinical significance and indication of management/referral route

Skin changes in the at-risk foot	Examples of associated medical disorder or abnormality. Generalized peripheral state (area >5cm)	Associated with abnormality or medical disorder. Discrete lesions, or affected area (area <5cm)	Clinical significance and possible clinical management
Surface texture			
Dry scaly (anhydrotic, may be with dry fissures)	Systemic sclerosis, ichthyosis, lymphoedema	Dermatological conditions (eg. psoriasis, contact dermatitis) skin infection (eg. tinea pedis [vesicular form], post bacterial infection warts)	May need to observe over a few days or ask patient/carer to observe, or refer to GP, dermatologist, state registered chiropodist/podiatrist (SRCh), specialist nurse, promptly or with less urgency depending on severity, history and provisional diagnosis. If wart is pain-free consider no intervention and advise accordingly
Thin, shiny (atrophic, may be with dry fissures)	Oedema, as above	Old blister/burn site, oedema (sausage toes), necrobiosis lipoidica (associated with diabetes)	May need to observe over a few days or ask patient/carer to observe, or refer to GP, dermatologist, state registered chiropodist/podiatrist (SRCh), specialist nurse promptly or with less urgency depending on history and provisional diagnosis. Ensure footwear is large enough for increasing oedema as day progresses
Macerated (white, soggy — may be interdigital, or any other site)	Over-hydration of skin	Lack of airflow between toes (may show wet fissures), pre-tissue breakdown, tissue break-down under intact epidermis	Check fit of footwear, toe function, dry between toes if uncomplicated maceration and astringe with, eg. surgical spirit. If pre- or overt-tissue breakdown, provide protective dressing and refer to GP, state registered chiropodist/podiatrist (SRCh), specialist nurse promptly
Hard and thickened skin	Associated with poor peripheral blood supply (eg. with diabetes, peripheral vascular disease), poor nutrition	Callus, corn (may be scar, [normal, hypertrophic or keloid]), gouty tophi, sclerosis (associated with eg. rheumatoid arthritis)	Refer to SRCh for treatment, or GP or specialist department
Tone			
Change in normal skin resilience (compared with contra lateral or more proximal site)	Oedema, collagen disorders (eg. systemic sclerosis rheumatoid arthritis), endocrine disorders (eg. myxoedema, diabetes)	Scarring (following single, or low grade repetitive trauma), inflammation (eg. bursitis), piezogenic papules	Observe over a few days-weeks and ask patient/carer to observe for changes from normal. Protect site with foam cushion pad if sufficient space in footwear. Refer to SCRCh, GP, specialist nurse for check-up, or treatment if condition appears to worsen
Smell (a tricky thing to assess)	Poor hygiene, food intake	Infection, fungating wound, poor hygiene, occlusive footwear	As for 'colour'

In dark-coloured skin some of the skin changes are less obvious and it is necessary to make careful observations.

No reference has been made to management of any medical condition in preference to outlining management of foot problems, and that information relates to those practitioners who feel they do not have the knowledge, skills or facilities to treat the problem.

Please note that this is not a definitive list, and should be used as guidance to direct further reading.

Index

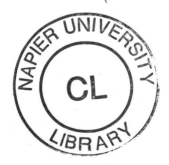